LIBRARY/NEW ENGLAND INST. OF TECHNOLOGY

D1563257

RM 300 .F38

Feix, Jeff.

Pharmacology handbook for
the surgical technologist

Pharmacology Handbook

for the Surgical Technologist

NEW ENGLAND INSTITUTE OF TECHNOLOGY
LIBRARY

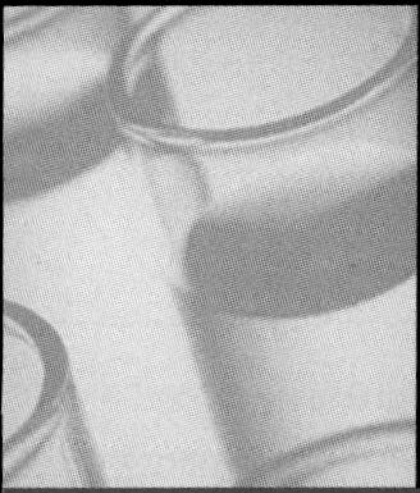

Pharmacology Handbook

for the Surgical Technologist

Second Edition

■ ■ ■

Jeff Feix, LVN, CST/CSFA, FAST

Surgical Technology Program

Coordinator/Instructor

Vernon College

Wichita Falls, Texas

NEW ENGLAND INSTITUTE OF TECHNOLOGY

LIBRARY

DELMAR

CENGAGE Learning™

Australia • Brazil • Japan • Korea • Mexico • Singapore • Spain • United Kingdom • United States

9-11

#727063857

DELMAR
CENGAGE Learning™

Pharmacology Handbook for the Surgical Technologist, Second Edition

Jeff Feix

Vice President, Editorial: Dave Garza

Director of Learning Solutions: Matt Kane

Executive Editor: Stephen Helba

Managing Editor: Marah Bellegarde

Senior Product Manager: Juliet Steiner

Editorial Assistant: Jennifer Wheaton

Vice President, Marketing: Jennifer Baker

Marketing Director: Wendy Mapstone

Senior Marketing Manager: Michele McTighe

Marketing Coordinator: Scott Chrysler

Production Director: Wendy Troeger

Production Manager: Andrew Crouth

Content Project Management: PreMediaGlobal

Senior Art Director: Jack Pendleton

© 2012, 2006 Delmar, Cengage Learning

ALL RIGHTS RESERVED. No part of this work covered by the copyright herein may be reproduced, transmitted, stored, or used in any form or by any means graphic, electronic, or mechanical, including but not limited to photocopying, recording, scanning, digitizing, taping, Web distribution, information networks, or information storage and retrieval systems, except as permitted under Section 107 or 108 of the 1976 United States Copyright Act, without the prior written permission of the publisher.

For product information and technology assistance, contact us at **Cengage Learning Customer & Sales Support, 1-800-354-9706**

For permission to use material from this text or product, submit all requests online at **www.cengage.com/permissions.** Further permissions questions can be e-mailed to **permissionrequest@cengage.com**

Library of Congress Control Number: 2011924554

ISBN-13: 978-1-111-30665-6

ISBN-10: 1-111-30665-6

Delmar
5 Maxwell Drive
Clifton Park, NY 12065-2919
USA

Cengage Learning is a leading provider of customized learning solutions with office locations around the globe, including Singapore, the United Kingdom, Australia, Mexico, Brazil, and Japan. Locate your local office at: **international.cengage.com/region**

Cengage Learning products are represented in Canada by Nelson Education, Ltd.

To learn more about Delmar, visit **www.cengage.com/delmar**

Purchase any of our products at your local college store or at our preferred online store **www.cengagebrain.com**

Notice to the Reader

Publisher does not warrant or guarantee any of the products described herein or perform any independent analysis in connection with any of the product information contained herein. Publisher does not assume, and expressly disclaims, any obligation to obtain and include information other than that provided to it by the manufacturer. The reader is expressly warned to consider and adopt all safety precautions that might be indicated by the activities described herein and to avoid all potential hazards. By following the instructions contained herein, the reader willingly assumes all risks in connection with such instructions. The publisher makes no representations or warranties of any kind, including but not limited to, the warranties of fitness for particular purpose or merchantability, nor are any such representations implied with respect to the material set forth herein, and the publisher takes no responsibility with respect to such material. The publisher shall not be liable for any special, consequential, or exemplary damages resulting, in whole or part, from the readers' use of, or reliance upon, this material.

Printed in China by China Translation & Printing Services Limited
1 2 3 4 5 6 7 15 14 13 12 11

Dedication

I would like to dedicate this book to my wife Joy for her understanding and support during the writing of this book. Researching and writing a project of this magnitude requires a significant amount of time away from family activities in the evening since I have another "regular" job during the day. Joy always provided words of encouragement and never complained of the many evenings she had to endure listening to me type away on my laptop.

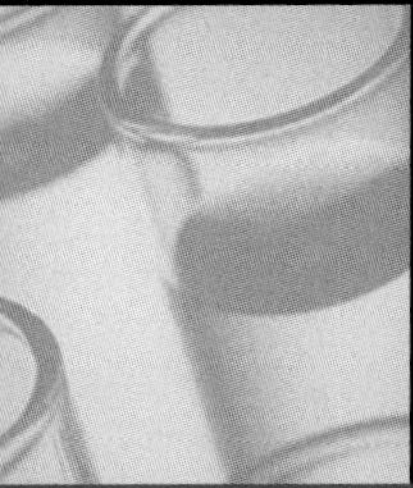

Contents

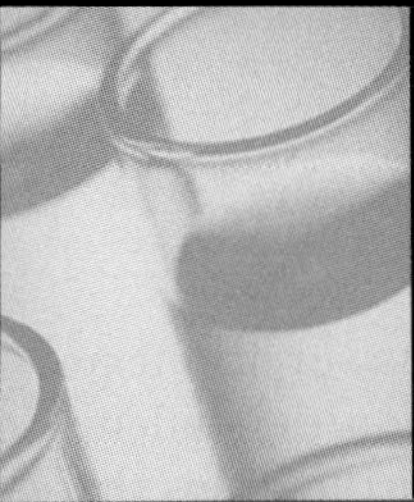

Preface

Pharmacology Handbook for the Surgical Technologist is designed to be a quick reference guide intended primarily for student surgical technologists, who will find this handbook most useful as a reference guide during their clinical rotation. When preparing for their surgical procedures, they can quickly check the "hard facts" about the drugs that will be involved and handled in the sterile field.

This handbook contains the most commonly used operating room drugs and is not intended to be used as a pharmacology textbook. The handbook contains terminology, abbreviations, a mathematics review, and drug cards. It was designed to incorporate objectives of the current edition of the Association of Surgical Technologists Core Curriculum in Education for Surgical Technology.

As a surgical technology educator, I found that the available pharmacology handbooks were designed for nurses with nursing considerations. In the observation clinical, my students had difficulty locating information for the drug cards that I required them to write, especially the anesthesia drugs used. When participating as surgical team members and preparing for procedures, students lacked a quick reference guide for the drugs that were being prepared or used. The latest edition of the Core Curriculum in Education for Surgical Technology requires students to be knowledgeable about drugs that surgical technologists do not necessarily handle, such as anesthetics and narcotics.

I designed this handbook to be small enough for students to carry to clinical rotations in their lab coat and quickly access information about the drugs used. Surgical technologists in some facilities have more drug-handling responsibilities, such as mixing or reconstituting drugs, so a section is included to serve as a quick reference to review the skills needed for this task.

ORGANIZATION

This handbook begins with basic review information that can be accessed easily and quickly on the job and in your training.

Section I: Common Terms and Abbreviations provides a terminology section to aid you in understanding drug company inserts about the drugs. The terminology section also serves as a review and includes commonly used abbreviations.

Section II: Principles of Pharmacology provides a basic review of information important to professional practice for the surgical technologist.

Section III: Practice of Pharmacology includes essential review information about medication administration and contains illustrations that are useful to review before handling drugs. A mathematics review is also provided to help with dosage calculations.

Section IV: Drug Reference Cards presents a list of 18 types of drugs the surgical technologist will commonly encounter. Each drug profile provides the basic information needed to handle drugs in the operating room and to understand the effects that drugs have on the human body.

FEATURES

- Unique drug pages contain drug name and classification, the action of the drug, the usual route of administration, storage and handling responsiblities, and contraindications in quick reference format.
- An essential terminology and abbreviation section is included for review.
- A mathematics review is provided to assist with dosage calculations.

NEW TO THIS EDITION

- All drug cards are completely updated to reflect current practice.
- A new smaller size allows greater portability for surgical professionals and learners.
- Several new classifications of drugs are provided, including Anticholinergic-Antimuscarinic Drugs and Neuromuscular Blocking Agents.

- The Principles of Pharmacology section is updated to include the Six Rights of Medication Administration.
- The Practice of Pharmacology section is revised to offer a more concise review of essential concepts.

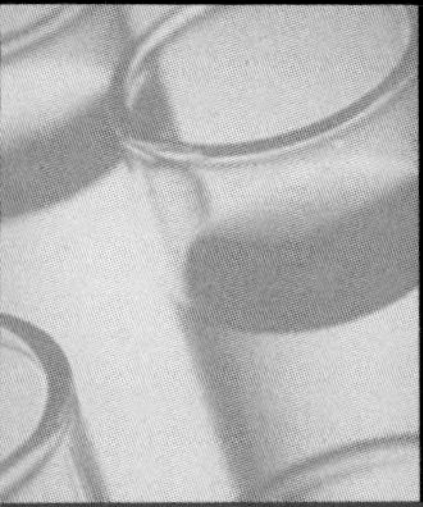

Reviewers

Sandra Berch, RN, BSN, CNOR
Indian River Community College
Port St. Lucie, Florida

Mercedes N. Alafriz Gordon
High-Tech Institute, Inc., The Bryman School
Phoenix, Arizona

Dana Grafft, CST
Iowa Lakes Community College
Spencer, Iowa

Jane Klick, RN, CNOR
Health Occupations Center
Columbia, Missouri

Rebecca Pieknik, CST, BHS
Oakland Community College and William Beaumont Hospital
Royal Oak, Michigan

Fred Valdes, MD
City College
Fort Lauderdale, Florida

Patti Ward, CST
Sanford Brown Institute
Jacksonville, Florida

Katherine J. Wolfer, RN, BSN, CNOR
Cincinnati State Technical and Community College
Cincinnati, Ohio

Roy Zacharias
Concorde Career Institute
Arlington, Texas

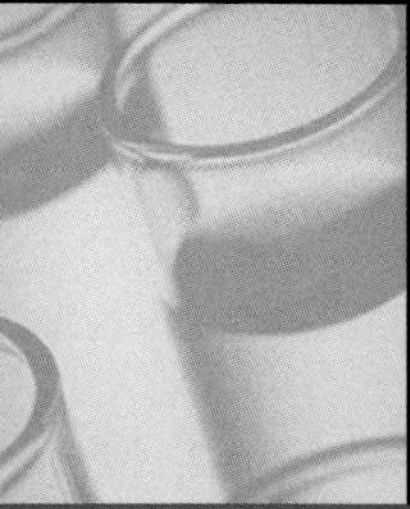

About the Author

Jeff Feix has been the Surgical Technology Coordinator/Instructor at Vernon College in Wichita Falls, Texas since 2002. He has been a surgical technology educator since 1999, starting his career as a surgical technologist in 1993. His credentials include the following:

- Licensed Vocational Nurse
- Certified Surgical Technologist
- Certified Surgical First Assistant
- Fellow of the Association of Surgical Technologists

Jeff originally decided to write a handbook geared toward surgical technology students when he found that one did not exist. Since the first edition was published he has found that many students continue to use this handbook after graduation when they begin work in the operating room. The new edition has been created with feedback from students, educators, and practitioners and incorporates their suggestions for improvement in the handbook.

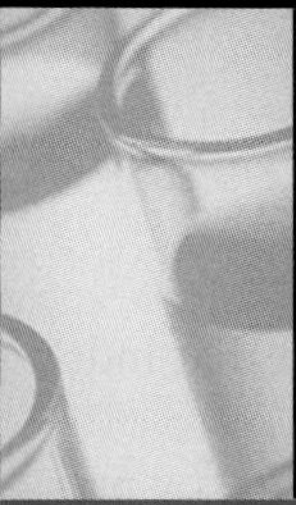

Section 1

Common Terms and Abbreviations

TERMINOLOGY

Absorption — the process of a drug passing through a body surface to the tissues of the body.

Action — a description of the cellular changes that occur as a result of a drug.

Adverse effects — possible untoward secondary effect other than the desired effect.

Adverse reaction — harmful unintended reactions to a drug.

Allergic reaction — hypersensitivity to a drug with symptoms ranging from a rash to an anaphylaxis.

Ampule — glass container for injectable drugs that must be broken at the neck to withdraw the medication.

Anaphylaxis — severe life-threatening hypersensitivity to a foreign substance or drug; symptoms include dyspnea, chest pain or tightness, life-threatening arrhythmias, and death.

Antagonism — opposing action of a drug that decreases or cancels the effect of another drug.

Buccal — within the cheek.

Contraindication — condition or situation that indicates a drug should not be given.

Controlled substance — a drug that is controlled by prescription because of the potential for addiction or abuse.

Cumulative effect — an increased effect of drug action it accumulates in the body.

Distribution — circulation of a drug to the organs of the body after the drug is absorbed.

Dosage — amount of drug given for the desired effect.

Generic name — general, common, or nonproprietary name of a drug.

Homeostasis — body in normal, balanced state.

Indication — condition that a drug is intended to treat.

Inhalation — the process of anesthesia by which an anesthetic gas is inhaled; some respiratory drugs also are inhaled as their route of administration.

Intra-articular — injected into the joint.

Intradermal (ID) — injected into layers of the skin.

Intramuscular (IM) — injected into a muscle.

Intravenous (IV) — injected in the vein.

Local (anesthetic) — medication administered to produce temporary loss of sensation or feeling in a specific area.

Parenteral — any route of administration not involving the gastrointestinal tract.

Placebo — medication with inert or inactive ingredients given in blind drug studies with no chemical effect on the patient. Used to measure effectiveness of the "real" drug being studied by comparing patients who take the placebo and patients who take the real drug.

Potentiation — increased effect when two drugs are given simultaneously for greater action than if given separately; also known as synergism.

Precautions — list of conditions or types of patients that require closer monitoring for specific side effects when given a drug.

Route — the specific method of delivery of a drug: PO, IM, IV, etc.

Subcutaneous (SC, SQ, SubQ) — beneath the skin.

Sublingual (SL) — under the tongue.

Topical — applied to a specific area for local effect, usually the skin or mucous membranes.

Toxicity — condition that occurs when a dangerous amount of a drug is given and that can be fatal depending on the drug and body systems affected.

Trade name (brand name) — name assigned to a drug by a pharmaceutical company.

Vial — glass or plastic container with a rubber stopper that must be punctured with a needle to withdraw a drug or reconstitute a drug in powder form.

ROUTES OF ADMINISTRATION

GI TRACT ROUTES

PO, or by mouth, the oral route to the gastrointestinal tract; the medication is absorbed in the stomach or intestines.

NG, or nasogastric tube, a tube inserted through the nose into the stomach. Special considerations should be observed when administering medications via this route to ensure proper placement of the NG tube in the stomach.

R, or rectally, medication is inserted into the rectum and absorbed by a rich network of capillaries.

PARENTERAL ROUTE—ANY ROUTE OTHER THAN GI

SL, or sublingual, medication is placed under the tongue and absorbed immediately into the circulatory system via the capillaries.

Buccal medication is placed between the cheek and gum and absorbed similar to sublingual.

INJECTION ROUTES

IV, or intravenous, medication is injected either directly into the vein or via an intravenous tube inserted into a vein or artery.

IM, or intramuscular, medication is injected into a muscle.

SubQ, or subcutaneous, medication is injected under the first layer of the skin.

ID, or intradermal, medication is injected in between the layers of the skin.

Intracardiac is when medication is injected directly into the heart.

Intra-articular is when medication is injected into a joint.

Intraspinal or **Intrathecal** medication is injected into the subarachnoid space, usually for epidural or spinal anesthesia.

OTHER

Topical medication is applied directly on skin or mucous membranes and absorbed in the capillaries.

Inhalation medication is inhaled into the lungs and absorbed into the circulatory system.

ABBREVIATIONS

bid — twice a day.
cc — cubic centimeters. (Joint Commission recommends accredited organizations replace cc with mL for milliliters.)
dc — discontinue.
g, gm — grams.
gt, gtt — drop(s).
HS — bedtime. (Joint Commission suggests writing out "at bedtime" so as not to confuse with half-strength.)
ID — intradermal.
IM — intramuscular.
IV — intravenous.
KVO — keep vein open.
mEq — milliequivalents.
mg — milligrams.
mL — milliliters.
NKA — no known allergies.
NPO — nothing by mouth.
PO — by mouth.
prn — as needed.
qid — four times a day.
R — rectal.
sub-Q, subQ — subcutaneous.
SL — sublingual.
stat — immediately.
T, tbs, tbsp — tablespoon.
t, tsp — teaspoon.
tid — three times a day.
X — times.

GENERAL DRUG CLASSIFICATIONS

Analeptics — drugs used to stimulate the central nervous system.

Analgesics — drugs used to relieve pain.

Anesthetics — drugs used to provide anesthesia for surgical procedures; can be delivered by local, regional, or general methods.

Antibiotics — drugs used to treat infection.

Anticoagulants — drugs used to reduce clotting factors of blood.

Anticonvulsants — drugs used to reduce and/or stop seizures/convulsions.

Antidiuretics — drugs used to decrease the excretion of urine.

Antiemetics — drugs used to prevent nausea and vomiting.

Cardiac medications — drugs used to increase or decrease heart function.

CNS Stimulants — drugs used to stimulate nerve receptors within the central nervous system.

Coagulants — drugs used to increase clotting factors of blood.

Contrast media — agents used to enhance visualization of anatomical structures and any abnormalities.

Diuretics — drugs used to increase the excretion of urine.

Dyes — drugs used to stain pathological specimens.

Emetics — drugs used to induce vomiting.

Gastric medications — drugs used to reduce secretions in the stomach.

Hemostatic agents — chemical agents in a variety of forms that enhance clot formation.

Hormones — drugs used to replace natural hormones usually produced in the body.

Irrigation solutions — fluids used to flush, wash, or soak structures/tissues during surgery.

Narcotic antagonists — drugs used to reverse the effects of narcotics.

Narcotics — drugs with a high potential for abuse.

Neuromuscular Blocking Agents—drugs used to relax skeletal muscles during surgery.

Obstetrical agents — drugs used during labor and childbirth.

Ophthalmic medications — drugs used in the eye.

Sedative/Hypnotic agents — drugs used to produce sedation or sleep.

Tranquilizers — drugs used to produce relaxation.

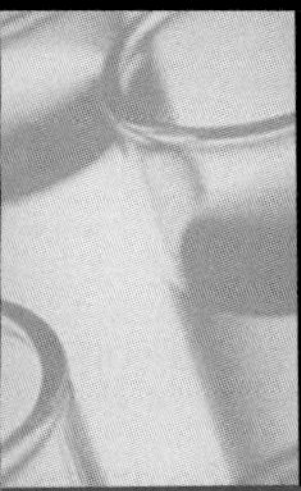

Section 2

Principles of Pharmacology

PHARMACOKINETICS

Pharmacokinetics, in simple terms, is when the body processes a drug. Once within the body, the drug undergoes several changes to include absorption, distribution, metabolism, and excretion.

Absorption is the drug getting into the bloodstream. Rate of absorption depends on method of administration; IV drugs are absorbed almost instantly while PO drugs may take 20 to 30 minutes to reach the bloodstream.

Distribution is the drug moving from the bloodstream into the tissues, fluids, and organs of the body. The chemical properties of the drug will determine the rate of distribution and the target cells or tissues for the desired effect.

Metabolism (biotransformation) is the physical and chemical changes that occur as the liver breaks down the drug and prepares it for excretion from the body. Some drugs can bypass the process of metabolism and reach the kidneys virtually unchanged. The rate of metabolism will depend on the drug as well as the patient's age, physical condition, and liver function.

Excretion is the process of the body removing the drug through the kidneys via urine. Some drugs can be excreted through the lungs, perspiration, feces, bile, and breast milk, but most are excreted by the kidneys.

VARIABLES AFFECTING PHARMACOKINETICS

Several variables can affect the speed and efficiency of the drug being processed by the body.

AGE

Older adults have slower metabolism and excretion rates; therefore, a cumulative effect can occur that may result in toxicity. Children have a lower threshold of response and react more rapidly and sometimes in unexpected ways.

WEIGHT

Generally the more a patient weighs, the larger the dose given, but there is a great variation in individual sensitivity to drugs and a manufacturer's instructions should be followed. Pediatric doses are usually calculated by weight.

SEX

Women and men may respond differently to the same drugs, and this may be due to hormones and ratio of body fat. Women who are pregnant or nursing usually have dosages adjusted or the drug is contraindicated.

PSYCHOLOGICAL STATE OF MIND

This variable is usually referred to as the placebo effect; the more positive a patient feels about a medication, the more positive the physical response.

PHYSICAL CONDITION

If the liver or kidneys are damaged by disease or trauma, drugs may not be metabolized properly and/or excreted properly. If the patient is immunocompromised, some drugs may have an untoward effect or no effect at all on target cells. Vascular disease or circulatory insufficiency can prevent the drugs from being distributed to target cells.

WRONG ROUTE OR INCORRECT ADMINISTRATION

Not administering drug as recommended can have life-threatening effects with some medications. Some oral drugs can be affected by meals and the pH level of the stomach. Medication errors occur due to human errors stemming from lack of attention to the six rights of medication administration.

SIX RIGHTS OF MEDICATION ADMINISTRATION

RIGHT PATIENT

The first step before administering any medication is ensuring that the correct patient is given the medication. Comparing the chart and/or order to the patient's ID bracelet and asking the patient to state his or her name can accomplish this task.

RIGHT MEDICATION

The drug label should be checked to ensure the correct medication is on hand. This label should be compared to the order sheet/chart to ensure the right medication is being administered. Always check the expiration date on the label as well. In the operating room all medications must be labeled immediately following their transfer to the sterile field.

RIGHT AMOUNT OR DOSE

The correct dosage is extremely important as many drugs can have life-threatening effects if administered in an incorrect dose, especially an overdose. In the operating room the surgeon's preference card will usually list the amount he or she wants on hand. It is the surgical technologist's responsibility to verify the dose with the surgeon and to know what amount of the drug can be given safely.

RIGHT TIME

Timing can be as important as dosage. Some medications have a cumulative effect that if given too close together can result in a life-threatening situation. Some local anesthetics may only be used for a specified amount of time. Always check to see if there is a time factor involved with the drugs being used.

RIGHT ROUTE

The correct route of administration is critical to the medication's efficiency and effectiveness. The surgical technologist should always be aware of the correct route to use medications in the field by correctly labeling medications, such as contrast media and local anesthetics such as lidocaine.

RIGHT DOCUMENTATION

Upon administration of medication, documentation in the patient's chart is required. This documentation should be done immediately upon administration as to the medication given, time, route, and by whom. Current state laws require a licensed nurse or certified medication aide to administer and document medications given. The surgical technologist is responsible to keep track of the amount of a drug used during the surgical procedure. This should be reported to the circulating Registered Nurse upon completion of the surgical procedure to be documented in the operative record.

PHARMACODYNAMICS

Pharmacodynamics is the term used to describe the interaction of the drug with the target cells.

Onset is the beginning of the drug's desired effect on the target cells within the body.

Peak (effect) is when the drug is at the most effective stage of the desired effect in the target cells.

Duration is the length of time between the onset of action and the cessation of action.

Indication is the condition or symptom in the patient that the drug is intended to treat or alleviate.

Contraindication is a condition or situation in which a drug should not be given. It can range from a hypersensitivity to the drug or another medication being taken, the combination of which could cause untoward effects.

Action is the effect of the drug at the target cells.

Side effects are secondary effects and are not the desired effect of the drug. Some side effects can be mild, such as a dry mouth, or more problematic, such as constipation. Generally, side effects are tolerated as they are usually mild.

Adverse effects are secondary effects that are more severe than side effects. Adverse effects can be life-threatening, such as an anaphylactic reaction or liver damage. When adverse effects are encountered, the medication is discontinued.

Tolerance is the reduced therapeutic response to a drug following repeated doses.

MEDICATION EFFECTS

Relaxation — desired effect is muscle relaxation; working on CNS receptors, nerve impulses are blocked to stop or delay muscle spasms.

Sedation — desired effect is calmness and decrease of nervousness to the point of the patient being induced to a state of sleep.

Amnesia — desired effect of IV conscious sedation agents and adjuncts to anesthesia in which the patient does not remember the immediate preoperative phase.

Neuroleptic — desired effect is tranquilizing action.

Analgesia — desired effect is to relieve pain; may be narcotic or nonnarcotic.

Drying agents — desired effect is to inhibit the secretion of fluids, usually in the respiratory tract.

Gastric acid reduction — desired effect is to reduce or inhibit gastric (stomach) secretions during all phases of surgery and postoperatively.

Vagal blockade — desired effect is to block stimulus to the vagus nerve, part of the autonomic nervous system.

MEDICATION ACTIONS

Synergist — an action that occurs when an agent increases the effectiveness of another agent that is combined with it.

Agonist — a chemical or drug action that occurs naturally in the body.

Antagonist — an action on the nervous system that occurs when a chemical or drug blocks the effect of a chemical or drug occurring naturally in the body (agonist) by combining with and blocking the agonist nervous receptor.

Additive — an action that occurs when a second agent is added to enhance the effect of the first agent.

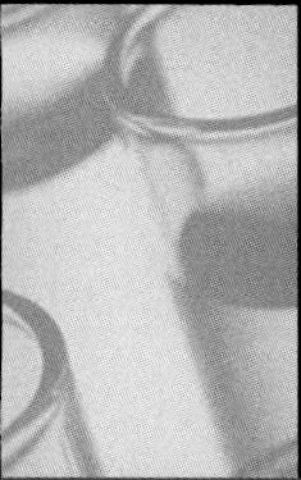

Section 3

Practice of Pharmacology

MEDICATION IDENTIFICATION

IDENTIFICATION—READING DRUG LABELS

Drug labels should be checked each time a drug is used. The drug label contains information that must be known before the medication is introduced onto the sterile field.

Critical elements that must be identified on the label are:

- Name of the drug
- Dosage or strength of the drug
- Correct form of the drug
- Expiration date of the drug
- Handling/storage instructions

NAME OF THE DRUG

Note the name of the drug in the following label (see Figure 3-1):
The name of the drug in Figure 3-1 is Robinul.

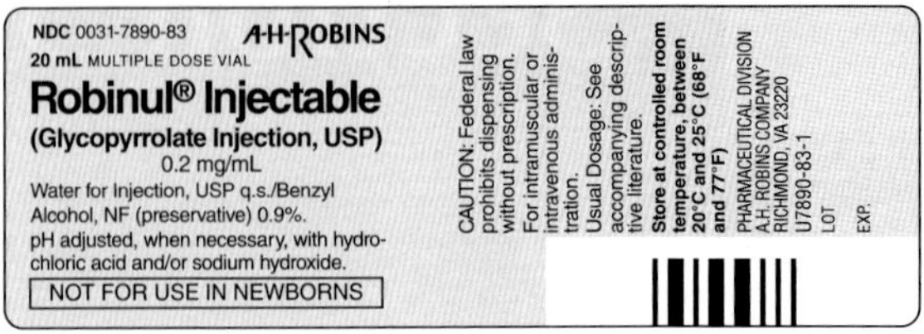

Courtesy of Baxter Health

FIGURE 3-1 **Robinul Injectable.**

DOSAGE OR STRENGTH OF THE DRUG

The strength of the drug in Figure 3-1 is 0.2 mg/mL.

FORM OF THE DRUG

In Figure 3-1, the drug is supplied in injection form.

EXPIRATION DATE OF THE DRUG

Note that the expiration date of the drug is printed on the drug's label.

MEDICATION MEASUREMENTS

The three primary systems to measure medications in the United States are the metric, household (U.S.), and apothecary systems of measurement.

METRIC SYSTEM

The metric system is a decimal system based on multiples of 10. The primary units of measurement are grams (g or gm) for weight, liters (L) for volume, and meters (m) for length. The system uses prefixes to determine the amount of the primary unit of measurement.

Micro — is one millionth or 0.000001 of the primary unit (micrograms or mcg).

Milli — is one thousandth or 0.001 of the primary unit (milligrams or mg).

Centi — is one hundredth or 0.01 of the primary unit (centimeters or cm).

Deci — is one tenth or 0.1 of the primary unit (deciliters or dl).

Kilo — is one thousand or 1000 times the primary unit (kilograms or kg).

WEIGHT

The gram is the primary or base unit of measurement.

1 g = 1000 mg
1 mg = 1000 mcg = 0.001 g
1 mcg = 0.001 mg = 0.000,001 g
1 kg = 1000 g

VOLUME

The liter is the primary or base unit of measurement.

1 L = 1000 mL
1 mL = 1 cc = 0.001 L
1 cc = 1 mL = 0.001 L

LENGTH

The meter is the primary or base unit of measurement.

1 m = 100 cm = 1000 mm
1 cm = 0.01 m = 10 mm
1 mm = 0.001 m = 0.1 cm

HOUSEHOLD SYSTEM

The household system is primarily used in the United States for home medication administration.

Drops (gtt)	Drop from a calibrated dropper	1gt = 0.05 mL
Teaspoon (t or tsp)	Common household teaspoon	1 tsp = 5 mL
Tablespoon (T or tbs)	Common household tablespoon	1 tbs = 15 mL
Ounce (oz) (fluid)		1 oz = 2 tbs = 30 mL
Ounce (oz) (weight)		1 pound (lb) = 16 oz = 500 mL
Cup		1 cup = 8 oz = 240 mL
Pint (pt)		1 pt = 2 cups = 500 mL
Quart (qt)		1 qt = 4 cups = 2 pt = 946.4 mL

APOTHECARY SYSTEM

The apothecary system is the original system of measurement for medications. It has been slowly phased out of use in the United States; however, a few hospitals still employ this system of measurement.

Grain (gr)	1 gr = 60 mg
Quart (qt)	1 qt = 2 pt

Pint (pt)	1 pt = 500 mL
Ounce (oz) or fluid dram	1 oz = 30 mL
Dram	1 dram = 4 g
Minim	1 minim = 1 drop

OTHER FORMS OF MEASUREMENT

- International unit is used to measure the potency of chemicals and vitamins.
- Unit is a standardized dose needed to produce a desired effect; insulin and heparin are examples.
- Milliunit is one thousandth of a unit.
- Milliequivalent (mEq) is one thousandth of an equivalent weight of a chemical and is used for calcium, potassium, magnesium, and sodium.

MEDICATION DELIVERY METHODS

PARENTERAL ADMINISTRATION

In the operating room, the majority of medications are delivered in IV form. This is the delivery method that will be illustrated.

All medications used in the sterile field must be labeled. Each syringe should be labeled, and any medication cup or sterile receptacle utilized should be labeled as well. The labels should be applied immediately after receiving, mixing, or drawing up the medication.

SYRINGES

Syringes are used to draw the medication from vials or ampules to mix or reconstitute the medication, inject medication in the IV solution, and irrigation. Syringes are available in a variety of measurements. Syringes either have a "slip tip" or luer lock tip that is used to attach to needles or IV tubing for administration. Increasingly, more syringes and IV administration tubing sets are being developed that do not require a needle. They are called needleless systems.

The basic components of the syringe are shown in Figure 3-2.

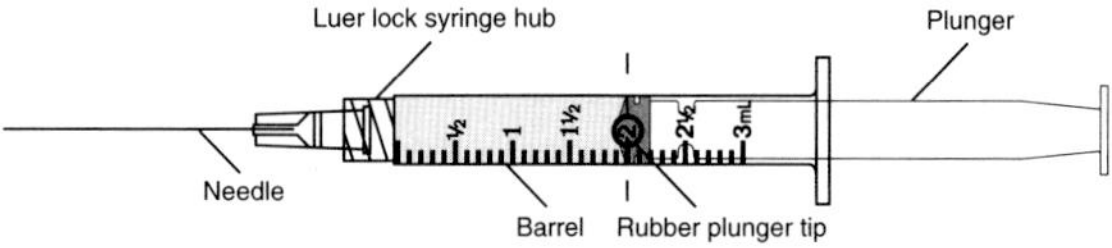

Delmar Cengage Learning

FIGURE 3-2 Syringe with needle unit.

When receiving the entire vial of a medication or when medication will be mixed, a medication cup should be used and labeled (see Figure 3-3). All drugs

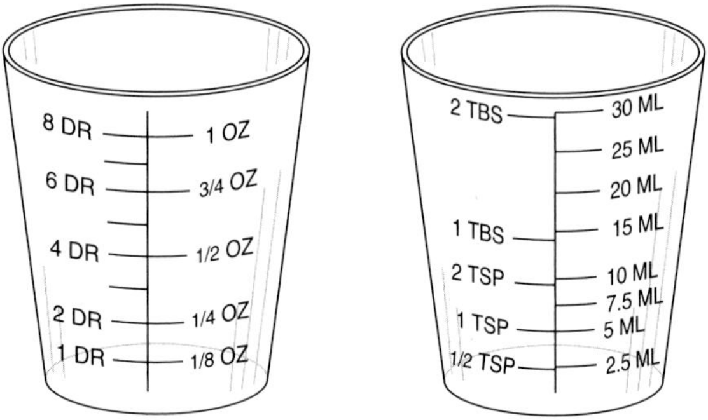

Delmar Cengage Learning

FIGURE 3-3 Medicine cups with approximate equivalent measures.

used in the sterile field must be labeled immediately upon receiving the drug.

STERILE AND NONSTERILE PREPARATION OF MEDICATION

IV forms of drugs are supplied in vials either in liquid form or powder form. The drug in powder form must be reconstituted with injectable Sterile Water or 0.9% injectable Sterile Saline. After the powder is completely dissolved, the medication is ready for use. IV forms of drugs are also supplied in ampules that require the top to be snapped off, and then the medication is withdrawn for use. Prefilled syringes are also available for some drugs. The various forms of delivery methods are shown in Figure 3-4.

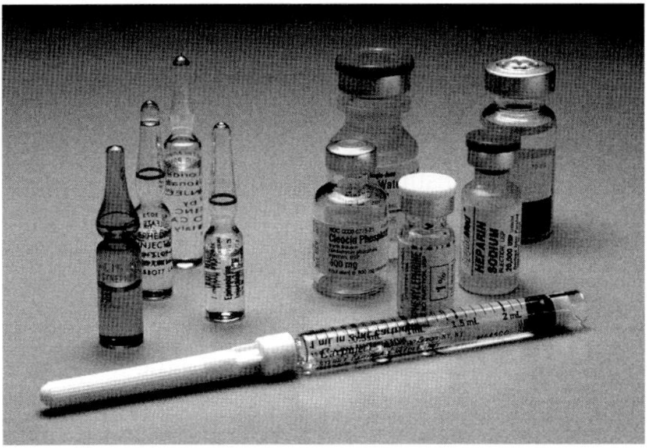

Delmar Cengage Learning

FIGURE 3-4 Ampules, vials, and a prefilled cartridge.

Medications are frequently mixed by the nonsterile circulating nurse and then given to the surgical technologist in a sterile fashion. On receiving medications, the surgical technologist is responsible for labeling syringes and medication cups that contain the drug. The name and strength of the medication should be repeated to the surgeon when passing the medications each time the drug is used.

NONSTERILE PREPARATION

Before preparing medications, wash and dry hands using aseptic technique.

Always verify that the drug to be used contains the correct name, dosage, and form, and then check the expiration date. The person who prepares the medication and the person receiving the medication should verify together these components before a drug is used. To prevent waste and for patient safety, the patient's allergies should be checked before preparation and use.

Most vial forms of medications have a plastic cap covering the rubber stopper; the cap will need to be removed to access the drug. Always use an alcohol pad to swab or wipe the top of the vial before withdrawing or reconstituting medications. Use a circular motion starting at the center and working out. Do not use bottled Saline/Sterile Water for reconstituting powder forms of drugs; only use injectable Sterile Water and Normal Saline. When reconstituting medications, always read the instructions on the drug label or insert.

The correct steps for reconstituting powder forms of IV drugs are shown in Figure 3-5.

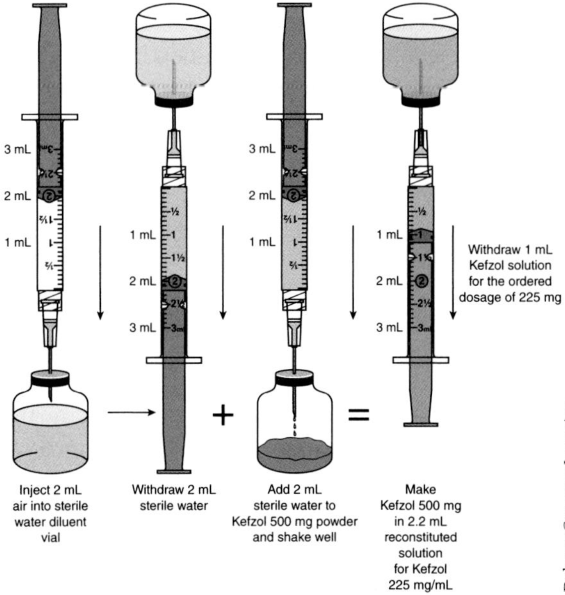
3 mL
2 mL
1 mL
Withdraw 1 mL Kefzol solution for the ordered dosage of 225 mg
Inject 2 mL air into sterile water diluent vial
Withdraw 2 mL sterile water
Add 2 mL sterile water to Kefzol 500 mg powder and shake well
Make Kefzol 500 mg in 2.2 mL reconstituted solution for Kefzol 225 mg/mL

Delmar Cengage Learning.

FIGURE 3-5 Procedure used for reconstituting powder forms of IV drugs.

When the medication is to be used in the sterile field, the circulator can pour the liquid form of the medication from the vial or use a syringe to inject it into a medication cup on the sterile field. When the drug must be reconstituted, the circulator can inject the medication from the syringe into a medication cup on the sterile field after preparing the drug.

When the drug is to be used in irrigation, the circulator should mix the medication into the

IV solution bag and then pour the solution with the aid of irrigation tubing. The medication can be injected into a bowl of injectable solution on the sterile field, but to ensure that the drug is adequately mixed it should be injected into the solution bag first, then the bag is gently shaken and the irrigation tubing inserted for introduction to the sterile field.

STERILE PREPARATION

Most drugs used in the sterile field will be introduced in liquid or IV form. Each drug, even if only one is used, must be labeled immediately when received on the sterile field. It is imperative that every medication cup and syringe on the sterile field be labeled with the name of the drug.

Since most drugs are introduced in liquid form, the sterile handling is relatively simple. A labeled medication cup should be used to accept the drug from the circulator. If used in irrigation, the circulator should mix before pouring the solution. In emergencies or procedures where an antibiotic irrigation is needed, the drug can be injected directly into IV solution in the sterile field. The surgical technologist should use an asepto syringe to mix the medication in the irrigation. When using irrigation with a medication such as an antibiotic, the surgical technologist should inform the surgeon of the drug in the irrigation.

When the medication is to be used "straight" or in undiluted form, the drug should be drawn from the medication cup into a syringe for use. The medication may be injected into tissue (a local anesthetic, for example) or it may be injected into an artery, as is the case with heparin, which is injected into an open artery/vein. The surgical technologist should prepare the syringe appropriately for use, ensuring that no air or air bubbles exist, and tell the surgeon the name and strength of the medication each time it is used. The surgical technologist should also keep track of the amount of each drug that is used and inform the circulator after the final count.

Other uses for drugs in the sterile field include soaking sponges or Gelfoam, soaking grafts, and some hemostatic agents, which require adding thrombin in liquid form to activate the agent.

MATHEMATICS REVIEW

The surgical technologist should have a basic knowledge of mathematics in order to ensure that the correct dosage, or amount of the drug, is being used. Since most drugs are supplied in the metric form and that system uses 10 as the base unit, most dosage conversions are straightforward. Conversions from the apothecary and household system are required occasionally, and conversion charts should be memorized or available for calculation.

EXAMPLE: The drug is supplied as 1 g in 10 mL and the surgeon wants to use 500 mg of the drug to mix with another medication.

How supplied:	1 g or 1000 mg in 10 mL
Dose needed:	500 mg
Calculation:	1000 mg ÷ 2 = 500 mg
	10 mL ÷ 2 = 5 mL
Amount to use:	5 mL of the drug will be needed.

EXAMPLE: The drug is supplied as 500 mg in 10 mL and the surgeon wants to use 2 g of the medication in an irrigation.

How supplied:	500 mg in 10 mL
Dose needed:	2 g or 2000 mg
Calculation:	500 mg × 4 = 2000 mg or 2 g
	10 mL × 4 = 40 mL
Amount to use:	40 mL of the drug will be needed.

EXAMPLE: The drug is supplied as 2.5 g in 5 mL and the surgeon wants to use 1.5 g.

How supplied:	2.5 g in 5 mL
Dose needed:	1.5 g
Calculation	2.5 g ÷ 5 = 0.5 g
	0.5 g × 3 = 1.5 g
Amount to use:	0.5 g/mL will require 3 mL.

Remember the following conversions and most of the calculations can be done mentally:

1 g = 1000 mg	1 g = 1.0 g
1/2 g = 500 mg	1/2 g = 0.5 g
1/4 g = 250 mg	1/4 g = 0.25 g

For medications that require a dosage calculation based on weight, the metric system uses kilograms instead of pounds. Remember 1 kg = 2.2 lb.

EXAMPLE: Patient weighs 150 lb

Calculation: 150 lb ÷ 2.2 = 68.18 kg

Patient weight for medication dosage calculation is 68 kg.

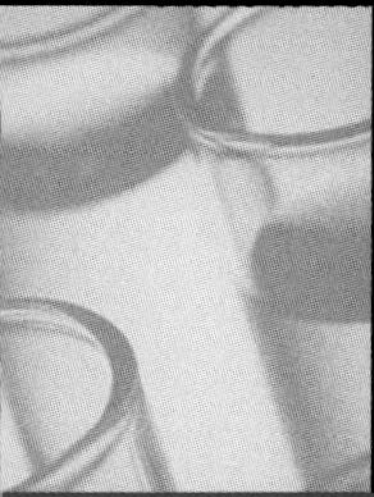

Section 4

Drug Reference Cards

ANALGESICS

alfentanil hydrochloride (Alfenta)

butorphanol tartate (Stadol)

fentanyl citrate (Sublimaze)

fentanyl and droperidol (Innovar)

hydromorphinone hydrochloride (Dilaudid)

ketorlac thromethamine (Toradol)

meperidine hydrochloride (Demerol)

morphine sulfate

nalbuphine hydrochloride (Nubain)

remifentanil hydrochloride (Ultiva)

sufentanil citrate (Sufenta)

alfentanil hydrochloride (Alfenta)

■ **Classification:** Analgesic (Narcotic)

HOW SUPPLIED/USUAL DOSAGE

Supplied in IV form and dosage is determined based upon its use and the patient's weight.

OR INDICATION/COMMON USE

Used as an adjunct for induction of general anesthesia, an anesthetic for intubation, and can be used in Monitored Anesthesia Care (MAC) as an analgesic agent.

CONTRAINDICATIONS

Should not be used in patients under 12 years of age.

SPECIAL CONSIDERATIONS

Respiratory depression and muscle rigidity are the most common side effects and can also cause nausea, hypotension, vomiting, confusion, and agitation.

butorphanol tartate (Stadol)

■ **Classification:** Analgesic (Narcotic)

HOW SUPPLIED/USUAL DOSAGE

IM/IV 1–2 mg every four hours

OR INDICATION/COMMON USE

Preoperatively for pain relief, intraoperative use as an adjunct to anesthesia, postoperatively for pain relief. Also used with patients in labor at full term and in early labor.

CONTRAINDICATIONS

Should not be used in patients with head injuries or increased intracranial pressure.

SPECIAL CONSIDERATIONS

Can cause drowsiness, dizziness, hypotension, bradycardia, respiratory depression, nausea, vomiting, and blurred vision.

fentanyl citrate (Sublimaze)

Classification: Analgesic (Narcotic)

HOW SUPPLIED/USUAL DOSAGE

IV/Regional—2–20 mcg/kg, General—150 mcg/kg

OR INDICATION/COMMON USE

Short-acting analgesic during operative and preoperative periods and as a narcotic supplement to general and regional anesthesia.

CONTRAINDICATIONS

Should not be used in patients with head injuries, increased cranial pressure, elderly, COPD and other respiratory problems, liver and kidney dysfunction, and bradycardic dysrhythmias.

SPECIAL CONSIDERATIONS

Can cause respiratory depression, nausea and vomiting, hypotension, sedation, and dizziness.

fentanyl and droperidol (Innovar)

Classification: Analgesic/Neuroleptic (Narcotic)

HOW SUPPLIED/USUAL DOSAGE

IV/Fentanyl .05 mg, Droperidol 2.5 mg

OR INDICATION/COMMON USE

Commonly used as an adjunct to anesthesia; resulting in an intense analgesic and amnesic state that may or may not cause unconsciousness. Effects often last up to six hours, resulting in effective pain control.

CONTRAINDICATIONS

Patients who have existing respiratory depression, hypotension, or bradycardia should not receive Innovar.

SPECIAL CONSIDERATIONS

Innovar does not have a toxic effect on the kidneys or liver and results in slight cardiac depression. Antiemetic effect occurs and can be used to treat pain/nausea.

hydromorphinone hydrochloride (Dilaudid)

■ **Classification:** Analgesic (Narcotic)

HOW SUPPLIED/USUAL DOSAGE

IM/IV 1–4 mg (slowly over 2 to 5 minutes) every 4 to 6 hours as needed.

OR INDICATION/COMMON USE

Postoperatively for moderate to severe pain relief.

CONTRAINDICATIONS

Should not be given to patients with decreased lung capacity, head injuries, and increased intracranial pressure.

SPECIAL CONSIDERATIONS

Care should be taken not to confuse Dilaudid with Dilantin or hydromorphinone with morphine. High potential for abuse/addiction, should not be used in patients with known drug addiction. Can cause dizziness, sedation, decreased respiratory, renal and bowel function, hypotension, bradycardia, nausea, vomiting, urinary retention, and blurred vision.

ketorlac tromethamine (Toradol)

■ **Classification:** Analgesic (NSAID, Non-Narcotic)

HOW SUPPLIED/USUAL DOSAGE

IM—60 mg or IV—30 mg every 6 hours.

OR INDICATION/COMMON USE

Postoperatively as mild to moderate pain relief.

CONTRAINDICATIONS

Should not be used in patients with a known hypersensitivity to NSAIDs, renal insufficiency, GI bleeding, active peptic ulcer disease, and risk of bleeding.

SPECIAL CONSIDERATIONS

Toradol is an excellent non-narcotic analgesic, but should not be used in surgical patients preoperatively or with patients who have a high risk of bleeding. Can cause drowsiness, headache, GI pain, urticaria, and pain at the injection site.

meperdine hydrochloride (Demerol)

■ **Classification:** Analgesic (Narcotic)

HOW SUPPLIED/USUAL DOSAGE

IM/IV 50–150 mg every 3 to 4 hours

OR INDICATION/COMMON USE

Preoperatively to produce relaxation, postoperatively for moderate to severe pain relief.

CONTRAINDICATIONS

Should not be given to patients with convulsive disorders or with undiagnosed abdominal pain.

SPECIAL CONSIDERATIONS

Can cause respiratory depression, dizziness, hypotension, nausea/vomiting, urinary retention, and urticaria.

morphine sulfate

■ **Classification:** Analgesic (Narcotic)

HOW SUPPLIED/USUAL DOSAGE

IV: 2.5–15 mg every four hours or 0.8–10 mg by continuous infusion. IM: 5–20 mg every four hours.

OR INDICATION/COMMON USE

Used pre- and postoperatively for relief of severe acute and chronic pain.

CONTRAINDICATIONS

Should not be given to patients with increased intracranial pressure, convulsive disorders, chronic pulmonary diseases, respiratory depression, undiagnosed abdominal pain, severe liver or kidney insufficiency, hypothyroidism, or following biliary tract surgery and surgical anastomosis.

SPECIAL CONSIDERATIONS

Can cause respiratory depression, hypotension, bradycardia, drowsiness, dizziness, urinary retention, and urticaria.

nalbuphine hydrochloride (Nubain)

■ **Classification:** Analgesic (Narcotic)

HOW SUPPLIED/USUAL DOSAGE

IM/IV 10–20 mg every 3 to 6 hours as needed. Maximum of 160 mg per day.

OR INDICATION/COMMON USE

Preoperatively as sedation/analgesia and as an adjunct to anesthesia. Postoperatively to relieve moderate to severe pain.

CONTRAINDICATIONS

Should not be given to patients with a known hypersensitivity.

SPECIAL CONSIDERATIONS

Can cause dizziness, drowsiness, nausea, vomiting, hypertension/hypotension, bradycardia/tachycardia, and blurred vision.

remifentanil hydrochloride (Ultiva)

■ **Classification:** Analgesic (Narcotic)

HOW SUPPLIED/USUAL DOSAGE

Supplied in IV form, and dosage is determined based upon its use as an adjunct to anesthesia or as an analgesic and also the patient's weight.

OR INDICATION/COMMON USE

Used as an analgesic agent during induction and maintenance of general anesthesia and as an analgesic during monitored anesthesia care.

CONTRAINDICATIONS

Should be administered only by anesthetists due to the potential apnea and respiratory depression associated with its use.

SPECIAL CONSIDERATIONS

Respiratory depression and apnea are associated with the administration of this drug. Ventilation and cardiac resuscitation should be readily available with its use.

sufentanil citrate (Sufenta)

■ **Classification:** Analgesic (Narcotic)

HOW SUPPLIED/USUAL DOSAGE

IV 1–8 mcg/kg as an analgesic supplement to anesthesia.
Primary anesthetic—1–30 mcg/kg administered with muscle relaxant IV and 100% oxygen.

OR INDICATION/COMMON USE

Used as a primary anesthetic and as an analgesic supplement in maintenance of balanced general anesthesia state.

CONTRAINDICATIONS

Pulmonary disease, reduced respiratory reserve, impaired hepatic, or renal function.

SPECIAL CONSIDERATIONS

Can cause hypotension/hypertension, bradycardia/tachycardia, nausea, vomiting, respiratory depression, apnea, skeletal muscle relaxant, and urinary retention.

ANESTHETICS

bupivacaine hydrochloride (Marcaine/ Sensorcaine)

Cetacaine

cocaine hydrochloride

Desflurane

droperidol (Inapsine)

Isoflurane

ketamine chloride (Ketalar)

lidocaine hydrochloride (Anestacon, Xylocaine)

methohexital sodium (Brevital Sodium)

mepivacaine hydrochloride (Carbocaine)

nitrous oxide

procaine hydrochloride (Novocain)

propofol (Diprivan)

Sevoflurane

tetracaine hydrochloride (Ponticaine)

thiopental sodium (Pentothal)

bupivacaine hydrochloride (Marcaine/Sensorcaine)

■ **Classification:** Anesthetic (Local/Regional)

HOW SUPPLIED/USUAL DOSAGE

Infiltration Anesthesia: IM-local infiltration sympathetic block 0.25% solution.
Epidural: Lumbar epidural 0.25%, 0.50%, and 0.75% solutions.
Caudal and peripheral block: 0.25% and 0.50% solutions.
Retrobulbar block: .075% solution.

OR INDICATION/COMMON USE

Local infiltration anesthesia, peripheral, sympathetic nerve, epidural including caudal block anesthesia. Commonly used forms include 0.5% to 1%. May be combined with epinephrine for enhanced effect and vasoconstriction at incision site.

CONTRAINDICATIONS

Should not be given to patients with acidosis, heart block, severe hemorrhage, hypotension, shock, cerebrospinal diseases, and a history of malignant hyperthermia.

SPECIAL CONSIDERATIONS

Can cause dizziness, urinary retention, hypotension, myocardial depression, bradycardia, nausea, vomiting, blurred vision, and pupillary constriction.

Cetacaine

Classification: Anesthetic (Topical)

HOW SUPPLIED/USUAL DOSAGE

Cetacaine is supplied in spray, liquid, and gel form, with the spray form being the most common OR use. Usual dose is a one-second spray for normal anesthesia.

OR INDICATION/COMMON USE

Typically used for endoscopic procedures in the ear, nose, mouth, larynx, pharynx, trachea, bronchi, and esophagus. Indicated for use in controlling gag reflex and pain when introducing flexible endoscopes orally.

CONTRAINDICATIONS

Should not be used in the eyes.

SPECIAL CONSIDERATIONS

Hypersensitivity is rare, and when using spray form any spray longer than two seconds is contraindicated.

cocaine hydrochloride

■ **Classification:** Anesthetic (Topical)

HOW SUPPLIED/USUAL DOSAGE

Topical: 1–10% solution with a maximum single dose of 1 mg/kg.

OR INDICATION/COMMON USE

Most common use is for topical anesthesia of the nose/throat.

CONTRAINDICATIONS

Should not be given to patients with a known hypersensitivity or sepsis in the region of application.

SPECIAL CONSIDERATIONS

Can cause CNS stimulation and depression, tachycardia, ventricular fibrillation, runny nose, nausea, and vomiting.

Desflurane

■ **Classification:** Anesthetic (Inhalation)

HOW SUPPLIED/USUAL DOSAGE

Supplied in colorless, non-flammable liquid form that utilizes a vaporizer for inhalation administration, and dosage is titrated to the patient's weight and other anesthetics agents being used. It produces a highly pungent odor.

OR INDICATION/COMMON USE

Used for induction and maintenance of general anesthesia and is typically mixed with oxygen, other inhalation agents, and frequently Sevoflurane for desired anesthetic effect.

CONTRAINDICATIONS

Should not be administered to patients with known hypersensitivity.

SPECIAL CONSIDERATIONS

Vaporizer should be calibrated and dosage calculated prior to administration. It has the most rapid onset and offset in effect of the inhalation agents. The use of opioids and benzodiazepines with Desflurane in surgical patients is common for the desired anesthesia effect.

droperidol (Inapsine)

■ **Classification:** Anesthetic Intravenous (Neuroleptic)

HOW SUPPLIED/USUAL DOSAGE

Premedication: IM/IV 2.5–10 mg 30–60 minutes preoperatively.
Maintenance of general anesthesia: IV 1.25–2.5 mg.

OR INDICATION/COMMON USE

Used for tranquilizing effect and to reduce nausea and vomiting, also as a premedication before induction of and the maintenance of general anesthesia.

CONTRAINDICATIONS

Should not be given to patients with a known hypersensitivity.

SPECIAL CONSIDERATIONS

Can cause postoperative drowsiness, dizziness, hypotension, tachycardia, and chills.

Isoflurane

■ **Classification:** Anesthetic (Inhalation)

HOW SUPPLIED/USUAL DOSAGE

Supplied in liquid form that utilizes a vaporizer for inhalation administration, and dosage is titrated to the patient's weight and other anesthetics agents being used. It is a clear, colorless, non-flammable liquid that produces a mildly pungent, musty ethereal odor.

OR INDICATION/COMMON USE

Used for induction and maintenance of general anesthesia and is typically mixed with oxygen, other inhalation agents, and nitrous oxide for desired anesthetic effect. In addition to anesthesia effect, Isoflurane has a muscle relaxant effect adequate for abdominal procedures.

CONTRAINDICATIONS

Should not be administered to patients with known hypersensitivity.

SPECIAL CONSIDERATIONS

Vaporizer should be calibrated and dosage calculated prior to administration. Respirations will rapidly decrease upon administration, and the patient will require respiratory support.

ketamine hydrochloride (Ketalar)

■ **Classification:** Anesthetic (Intravenous)

HOW SUPPLIED/USUAL DOSAGE

IV 1–4.5 mg/kg slowly over one minute

OR INDICATION/COMMON USE

Sole anesthetic agent for surgical procedures of short duration that do not require skeletal muscle relaxation. Can be used to induce anesthesia before administration of other general anesthetics or to supplement low-potency anesthetics.

CONTRAINDICATIONS

Should not be given to patients with severe hypotension, severe coronary disease, increased intracranial pressure, history of cerebrovascular injury, increased intraocular pressure, and surgery of the pharynx, larynx, and bronchial tree.

SPECIAL CONSIDERATIONS

Can cause hallucinations, delirium, muscular rigidity, increased intracranial pressure, hypertension, arrhythmias, mild increase in intraocular pressure, nausea, vomiting, respiratory depression, and laryngospasm.

lidocaine hydrochloride (Anestacon, Xylocaine)

- **Classification:** Anesthetic (Topical/Local/Regional), Antiarrhythmic

HOW SUPPLIED/USUAL DOSAGE

Infiltration Anesthesia: 0.50–1% solutions.
Nerve and epidural block: 1–2% solutions.
Caudal: 1–1.5% solutions.
Spinal: 5% with glucose.
Saddle block: 1.5% with dextrose.
Ventricular Arrhythmias: IV 50–100 mg bolus or at a rate of 20–50 mg/minute.
Supplied in gel form for topical use with oral endoscopy as a topical agent.

OR INDICATION/COMMON USE

Local and regional anesthetic and rapid control of ventricular arrhythmias. Commonly used forms include 0.5%, 1%, and 2% and may be combined with epinephrine added for an enhanced effect and vasoconstriction at the incision site.

CONTRAINDICATIONS

Patients with severe trauma or sepsis, arrhythmias, bradycardia, or heart block of any type.

SPECIAL CONSIDERATIONS

Can cause dizziness, difficult breathing or swallowing, hypotension, bradycardia, heart block, tinnitis, blurred vision, impaired color perception, nausea, vomiting, and excessive perspiration.

methohexital sodium (Brevital Sodium)

■ **Classification:** Anesthetic (Intravenous)

HOW SUPPLIED/USUAL DOSAGE

Induction of anesthesia: IV 5–12 mL of 1% solution at a rate of 1mL every 5 minutes and then 2–4 mL every 4 to 7 minutes as needed.

OR INDICATION/COMMON USE

Induction of anesthesia, as a supplement for other anesthetics, and as a general anesthetic for brief procedures.

CONTRAINDICATIONS

Should not be given to pregnant patients.

SPECIAL CONSIDERATIONS

Can cause severe respiratory and cardiovascular depression.

mepivacaine hydrochloride (Carbocaine)

■ **Classification:** Anesthetic (Local)

HOW SUPPLIED/USUAL DOSAGE

Infiltration Anesthesia: 0.50–1% Peripheral nerves 1–2%.
Maximum dose—500 mg.

OR INDICATION/COMMON USE

Local/regional anesthetic, including peripheral nerve block and epidural.

CONTRAINDICATIONS

Should not be given to patients with known hypersensitivity.

SPECIAL CONSIDERATIONS

Drug has few adverse effects and minimal tissue irritation.

nitrous oxide

■ **Classification:** Anesthetic (Inhalation)

HOW SUPPLIED/USUAL DOSAGE

Supplied in gas form, and dosage is titrated to the patient's weight and other anesthetics agents being used. It is a colorless non-flammable gas with a slight sweet taste and odor.

OR INDICATION/COMMON USE

Used as an inhalation agent in conjunction with other inhalants to produce analgesia and anesthesia effect for surgical procedures. It is an effective adjunct for induction and general anesthesia.

CONTRAINDICATIONS

Not indicated to be used as the sole anesthetic for large surgical procedures as it will not produce the analgesic effect required.

SPECIAL CONSIDERATIONS

Nitrous oxide is frequently called laughing gas and is used in dentistry as well.

procaine hydrochloride (Novocain)

■ **Classification:** Anesthetic (Local/Regional)

HOW SUPPLIED/USUAL DOSAGE

Infiltration anesthesia/Peripheral nerve block: 0.25–0.50% solution.

OR INDICATION/COMMON USE

Spinal anesthesia and epidural and peripheral nerve block by injection and infiltration methods.

CONTRAINDICATIONS

Should not be given to patients with heart block, hypotension, hypertension, and GI bleeding or hemorrhage.

SPECIAL CONSIDERATIONS

Can cause tinnitus, arrhythmias, hypotension, bradycardia, nausea, vomiting, sweating, and urinary retention in spinal anesthesia.

propofol (Diprivan)

■ **Classification:** Anesthetic (Intravenous)

HOW SUPPLIED/USUAL DOSAGE

Induction: IV 2–2.5 mg/kg every 10 seconds until induction onset.
Maintenance: IV 100–200 mcg/kg/minute.
Consciousness Sedation: IV 5 mcg/kg/minute for at least 5 minutes.

OR INDICATION/COMMON USE

Induction and/or maintenance of anesthesia.

CONTRAINDICATIONS

Should not be given to patients with a hypersensitivity to soybean oil or egg, increased intracranial pressure, impaired cerebral circulation, or any obstetric procedure.

SPECIAL CONSIDERATIONS

Can cause twitching, bucking, jerking, thrashing, hypotension, vomiting, coughing, and apnea. Drug will cause respiratory depression and is white in color.

Sevoflurane

Classification: Anesthetic (Inhalant)

HOW SUPPLIED/USUAL DOSAGE

Supplied in colorless, non-flammable liquid form that utilizes a vaporizer for inhalation administration, and dosage is titrated to the patient's weight and other anesthetics agents being used. Sevoflurane has a sweet-smelling odor and is used for mask anesthesia on adult and pediatric patients.

OR INDICATION/COMMON USE

Used for induction and maintenance of general anesthesia and is typically mixed with oxygen and inhalation agents for the desired anesthetic effect. Desflurane is most frequently used with Sevoflurane, and nitrous oxide is utilized for improved anesthetic effect.

CONTRAINDICATIONS

Should not be administered to patients with known hypersensitivity.

SPECIAL CONSIDERATIONS

Vaporizer should be calibrated and dosage calculated prior to administration. Respiratory support may be required with mask anesthesia, and airway should be maintained while administering Sevoflurane.

tetracaine hydrochloride (Ponticaine)

■ **Classification:** Anesthetic (Topical/Local/Regional)

HOW SUPPLIED/USUAL DOSAGE

Topical: Ophthalmic 1 to 2 drops of 0.5% solution.
Spinal: 1% solution diluted with equal volume of 10% dextrose injected in the subarachnoid space.

OR INDICATION/COMMON USE

Topical surface anesthesia in ophthalmic superficial procedures and also to paralyze laryngeal and esophageal reflexes prior to endoscopic procedures. Local infiltration and spinal anesthesia uses.

CONTRAINDICATIONS

Should not be given to patients with renal insufficiency, hypotension, bradycardia, or a known hypersensitivity.

SPECIAL CONSIDERATIONS

Ophthalmic solution should be instilled in lower conjunctival fornix. Spinal can be used high or low producing saddle block.

thiopental sodium (Pentothal)

■ **Classification:** Anesthetic (Intravenous)

HOW SUPPLIED/USUAL DOSAGE

Induction: IV test dose of 25–75 mg, then 50–75 mg at 20–40 second intervals.

OR INDICATION/COMMON USE

To induce hypnosis and anesthesia prior to or as a supplement to other anesthetic agents being used or as a sole agent for brief procedures.

CONTRAINDICATIONS

Should not be given to patients with asthma, hepatic disease, or a known hypersensitivity.

SPECIAL CONSIDERATIONS

Can cause severe myocardial and circulatory depression, retrograde amnesia, nausea, vomiting, regurgitation, respiratory depression, coughing, bronchospasm, laryngospasm, salivation, and skeletal muscle hyperactivity.

ANTIBIOTICS

ampicillin socium and sulbactam sodium (Unasyn)

aztreonam (Azactam)

bacitracin

cefaperazone sodium (Cefobid)

cefazolin sodium (Ancef, Kefzol)

cefotetan disodium (Cefotan)

cefoxitin sodium (Mefoxin)

ceftazidime (Fortaz)

cefuroxime sodium (Zinacef)

ciprofloxacin (Cipro IV)

co-trimoxazole (Bactrim, Bactrim DS)

gentamicin sulfate (Garamycin)

kanamycin (Kantrex)

metronidazole (Flagyl)

rocephin

vancomycin hydrochloride (Vancomycin)

ampicillin sodium and sulbactam sodium (Unasyn)

■ **Classification:** Antibiotic (Anti-infective)

HOW SUPPLIED/USUAL DOSAGE

IV 1.5 to 3 g mixed in 50 to 100 mL of Normal Saline every six hours.

OR INDICATION/COMMON USAGE

Typically is administered IV to treat intra-abdominal and gynecological infections but is also effective against staphylococcus aureus.

CONTRAINDICATIONS

Should not be administered with patients who have a known hypersensitivity to the drug or any of the penicillin family of drugs.

SPECIAL CONSIDERATIONS

Unasyn is an injectable antibacterial combination consisting of the semi-synthetic antibiotic ampicillin sodium and the beta-lactamase inhibitor sulbactam sodium for intravenous and intramuscular administration. Ampicillin sodium is derived from the penicillin nucleus.

aztreonam (Azactam)

■ **Classification:** Antibiotic (Anti-infective)

HOW SUPPLIED/USUAL DOSAGE

IV 0.5 to 2 g every 8 to 12 hours up to a maximum of 8 g/day.

OR INDICATION/COMMON USAGE

Used to treat infections of the urinary tract, lower respiratory tract, skin, soft tissue, female reproductive tract, intra-abdominal infections, septicemia, and surgical abscesses caused by gram-negative bacteria. Typically administered IV pre and postoperatively to treat infections and less often as prophylactic treatment.

CONTRAINDICATIONS

Should not be given to patients with known hypersensitivity or patients with impaired renal function.

SPECIAL CONSIDERATIONS

Can destroy normal flora, which requires monitoring the patient for possible post-treatment infections.

bacitracin

■ **Classification:** Antibiotic (Anti-infective)

HOW SUPPLIED/USUAL DOSAGE

IV—50,000 units in powder form for reconstitution
Also available as an ointment for topical use.

OR INDICATION/COMMON USE

Used primarily as a prophylactic in irrigation solution during surgical procedures.

CONTRAINDICATIONS

Should not be used in patients with a known hypersensitivity.

SPECIAL CONSIDERATIONS

When reconstituted and mixed in IV solution the drug will cause excessive bubbling, and this is a normal chemical reaction.

cefaperazone sodium (Cefobid)

■ **Classification:** Antibiotic (Cephalosporins)

HOW SUPPLIED/USUAL DOSAGE

IV—1 to 2 gm 30 minutes before surgery.

OR INDICATION/COMMON USE

Typically administered preoperatively in surgical procedures where risk for infection is high or the patient is currently infected and surgery cannot wait.

CONTRAINDICATIONS

Should not be given to patients with a known hypersensitivity to Cephalosporins.

SPECIAL CONSIDERATIONS

Should be given in diluted IV Normal Saline and may be given by IV piggyback or over 3 to 5 minutes IV bolus.

cefazolin sodium (Ancef/Kefzol)

■ **Classification:** Antibiotic (Cephalosporins)

HOW SUPPLIED/USUAL DOSAGE

IV—1 gm 30 to 60 minutes before surgery/1 gm diluted in 500 to 1000 mL Normal Saline.

OR INDICATION/COMMON USE

Typically the drug is administered IV for prophylactic effect before surgery and during contaminated procedures. It can also be used as a prophylactic in irrigation solution during surgical procedures.

CONTRAINDICATIONS

Should not be given to patients with a history of hypersensitivity to Cephalosporins.

SPECIAL CONSIDERATIONS

Should not be reconstituted with Lactated Ringers.

cefotetan disodium (Cefotan)

■ **Classification:** Antibiotic (Cephalosporins)

HOW SUPPLIED/USUAL DOSAGE

IV—1 to 2 gm 30 to 60 minutes before surgery.

OR INDICATION/COMMON USE

Typically the drug is administered IV preoperatively for prophylactic effect during surgery.

CONTRAINDICATIONS

Should not be given to patients with a hypersensitivity to Cephalosporins.

SPECIAL CONSIDERATIONS

If used during Caesarean section, dosage should not be administered until after the umbilical cord is clamped.

cefoxitin sodium (Mefoxin)

■ **Classification:** Antibiotic (Cephalosporins)

HOW SUPPLIED/USUAL DOSAGE

IV—1 to 2 gm injection or infusion.

OR INDICATION/COMMON USE

Typically is administered IV to treat serious infections of the respiratory, GI, GU tracts, or joints.

CONTRAINDICATIONS

Should not be given to patients with known hypersensitivity to Cephalosporins.

SPECIAL CONSIDERATIONS

Injection should be reconstituted with 10 mL of Sterile Water and given in a large vein over 3 to 5 minutes.

ceftazidime (Fortaz)

Classification: Antibiotic (Cephalosporins)

HOW SUPPLIED/USUAL DOSAGE

IV—1 to 2 gm injection or infusion.

OR INDICATION/COMMON USE

Typically is administered IV to treat serious infections of the lower respiratory tract, urinary tract, and intra-abdominal infections.

CONTRAINDICATIONS

Should not be given to patients with known hypersensitivity to Cephalosporins.

SPECIAL CONSIDERATIONS

Different manufacturers have specific and differing directions for reconstituting the drug, so follow label instructions closely.

cefuroxime sodium (Zinacef)

■ **Classification:** Antibiotic (Cephalosporins)

HOW SUPPLIED/USUAL DOSAGE

IV—1.5 gm 30 to 60 minutes preoperatively.

OR INDICATION/COMMON USE

Typically is administered IV for prophylactic effect prior to surgical procedure.

CONTRAINDICATIONS

Should not be given to patients with known hypersensitivity to Cephalosporins.

SPECIAL CONSIDERATIONS

If given by injection; give in large vein and deliver drug over 3 to 5 minutes.

ciprofloxacin (Cipro IV)

■ **Classification:** Antibiotic (Fluoroquinolones)

HOW SUPPLIED/USUAL DOSAGE

IV—400 mg.

OR INDICATION/COMMON USE

Typically is administered IV to treat mild to severe infections, including complicated and severe bone infections.

CONTRAINDICATIONS

Should not be given to patients with known hypersensitivity to Fluoroquinolones.

SPECIAL CONSIDERATIONS

IV infusion should be diluted with D5W or Normal Saline and infused slowly over one hour into a large vein.

co-trimoxazole (Bactrim, Bactrim DS)

Classification: Antibiotic (Sulfonamides)

HOW SUPPLIED/USUAL DOSAGE

IV—8 to 10 mg diluted in IV Normal Saline.

OR INDICATION/COMMON USE

Typically used for prophylactic effect in irrigation solution in a variety of specialties.

CONTRAINDICATIONS

The drug should not be used in surgical procedures with patients who have a known hypersensitivity to the drug or Sulfa. Should not be used when patient is pregnant or breast-feeding.

SPECIAL CONSIDERATIONS

If given by IV infusion, should be mixed according to label instructions and given over 60 to 90 minutes.

gentamicin sulfate (Garamycin)

■ **Classification:** Antibiotic (Aminoglycosides)

HOW SUPPLIED/USUAL DOSAGE

IV—1.5 mg/kg 30 minutes before surgery; maximum dose is 80 mg.

OR INDICATION/COMMON USE

Typically is administered IV for Endocarditis prophylaxis in GI or GU surgical procedures.

CONTRAINDICATIONS

Should not be given to patients with hypersensitivity to aminoglycosides.

SPECIAL CONSIDERATIONS

Observe urine output for possible decreased renal function.

kanamycin (Kantrex)

■ **Classification:** Antibiotic (Aminoglycosides)

HOW SUPPLIED/USUAL DOSAGE

IV—500 mg diluted in 500 to 1000 mL of Normal Saline.

OR INDICATION/COMMON USE

Typically is used for prophylactic effect in irrigation solution during GI or GU surgical procedures. Can be instilled via wound drain—500 mg diluted in 20 mL of Normal Saline for serious infections. Can also be administered IV for systemic prophylaxis as well.

CONTRAINDICATIONS

Should not be used with patients who have a known hypersensitivity to aminoglycosides.

SPECIAL CONSIDERATIONS

When used in irrigation solution during surgical procedures, IV Normal Saline should be used.

metronidazole (Flagyl)

■ **Classification:** Antibiotic (Amebicide)

HOW SUPPLIED/USUAL DOSAGE

IV—15mg/kg infusion over 30 to 60 minutes pre-operatively.

OR INDICATION/COMMON USE

Typically is administered IV for prophylactic effect before colorectal surgical procedures.

CONTRAINDICATIONS

Should not be given to patients with hypersensitivity to the drug.

SPECIAL CONSIDERATIONS

Do not give IV bolus of drug; it must be diluted in at least 100 mL of Lactated Ringers or Normal Saline.

rocephin

Classification: Antibiotic (Cephalosporins)

ANTIBIOTICS

HOW SUPPLIED/USUAL DOSAGE

IV—1 to 2 gm injection or infusion.

OR INDICATION/COMMON USE

Typically is administered IV to treat most infections and serious intra-abdominal infections.

CONTRAINDICATIONS

Should not be given to patients with known hypersensitivity to Cephalosporins.

SPECIAL CONSIDERATIONS

If administered by IM injection; should be given in large muscle and Lidocaine, or another topical anesthetic, can be diluted with the drug to reduce pain at the injection site.

vancomycin hydrochloride (Vancomycin)

■ **Classification::** Antibiotic (Anti-infective)

HOW SUPPLIED/USUAL DOSAGE

Powder 500 mg to 1 gm for IV infusion. Usually 1 to 1.5 gm IV every 12 hours.

OR INDICATION/COMMON USE

Typically is administered IV to treat serious or severe infections when other antibiotics are ineffective or contraindicated. The antibiotic of choice used to treat MRSA, though some strains have developed that are Vancomycin resistant. In some regions Vancomycin is used as a prophylactic treatment in total joint replacement procedures being administered at least one hour prior to the start of the procedure.

CONTRAINDICATIONS

Should not be given to patients with known hypersensitivity to the drug.

SPECIAL CONSIDERATIONS

Powder should be reconstituted with D5W or Normal Saline and infused over 60 minutes. If dose is greater than 1.5 gm, should be given over 90 minutes.

ANTICHOLINERGIC/ ANTIMUSCARINIC

atropine sulfate

glycopyrrolate (Robinul)

atropine sulfate

Classification: Anticholinergic/Antimuscarinic

HOW SUPPLIED/COMMON DOSAGE

IV injection with an adult dose of 0.4 to 0.6 mg given preoperatively and a pediatric dose 0.01 mg/kg up to a total of 0.4 mg given preoperatively.

OR INDICATION/COMMON USE

Given preoperatively to reduce respiratory tract secretions and facilitate intubation. Can also be given IV to treat bradycardia.

CONTRAINDICATIONS

Should not be given to patients with known hypersensitivity and who have angle-closure glaucoma. Should not be given to patients experiencing tachycardia.

SPECIAL CONSIDERATIONS

Used preoperatively for drying of secretions prior to surgery and anesthesia. Can be combined with sedatives and used as a preoperative adjunct to calm the pediatric patient and dry secretions.

glycopyrrolate (Robinul)

Classification: Anticholinergic

HOW SUPPLIED/USUAL DOSAGE

IV injection and can be given as IM injection also. IV adult dose 4.4 mcg/kg 30 to 60 minutes preoperatively not to exceed 0.1 mg. IV pediatric dose 4.4 to 8.8 mcg/kg 30 to 60 minutes preoperatively.

OR INDICATION/COMMON USE

Given preoperatively to reduce respiratory tract secretions and facilitate intubation.

CONTRAINDICATIONS

Should not be given to patients with known hypersensitivity and who have angle-closure glaucoma.

SPECIAL CONSIDERATIONS

Used preoperatively for drying of secretions prior to surgery and anesthesia. Can be combined with sedatives and used as a preoperative adjunct to calm the pediatric patient and dry secretions.

ANTICOAGULANTS

heparin calcium/heparin sodium

streptokinase (Kabikinase, Streptase)

heparin calcium/heparin sodium

■ **Classification:** Anticoagulant

HOW SUPPLIED/USUAL DOSAGE

Injection form supplied in vials of varying unit dosages depending upon manufacturer, with the usual or standard being 5000 units per 1 mL. Also supplied in syringe form. Surgeon or anesthesia usually determine dosage used based upon the procedure being performed.

OR INDICATION/COMMON USE

Used in surgery for prevention of DVT, treatment of pulmonary embolism, during open heart and vascular procedures, and in irrigation for vascular procedures.

Used during carotid endarterectomy in irrigation and can be injected full strength directly into the artery. Used during declotting and insertion of grafts and vessels.

Typically given by anesthesia and must be allowed to circulate for three minutes before incising artery or vein being repaired/replaced.

CONTRAINDICATIONS

Should not be administered to patients with a history of hypersensitivity to the drug, active bleeding disorders, during brain, eye or spinal surgery, and ideally not during spinal anesthesia.

(continues)

heparin calcium/heparin sodium continued

SPECIAL CONSIDERATIONS

Onset is considered to be immediate when given IV, but standard of care is to wait three minutes after anesthesia infuses drug before incising artery or vein. During procedures lasting four to six hours heparin is usually repeated since the actual duration during the procedure varies based on the dosage administered. During open-heart procedures a coagulant is given to reverse the effects of heparin.

streptokinase (Kabikinase, Streptase)

■ **Classification:** Anticoagulant

HOW SUPPLIED/USUAL DOSAGE

100,000 U to 250,000 U in 100—250 mL IV Normal Saline.

OR INDICATION/COMMON USE

Used in vascular procedures where thrombus is present. Commonly used in embolectomy and thrombectomy procedures to prevent thrombus formation postoperatively.

CONTRAINDICATIONS

Should not be used in patients with intracranial bleeding or active internal bleeding.

SPECIAL CONSIDERATIONS

Can be instilled into veins/arteries with small feeding tube and syringe.

ANTIEMETICS

droperidol (Inapsine)

metoclopramide hydrochloride (Reglan)

promethazine (Phenergan)

ondansetron hydrochloride (Zofran)

prochlorperazine (Compazine)

droperidol (Inapsine)

■ **Classification:** Antiemetic

HOW SUPPLIED/USUAL DOSAGE

IV 2.5 mg for adults.

OR INDICATION/COMMON USE

Used as an adjunct to general and regional anesthesia. Also used to reduce postoperative nausea and vomiting.

CONTRAINDICATIONS

Should not be given to patients with known hypersensitivity, narrow-angle glaucoma, and severe liver or cardiac disease.

SPECIAL CONSIDERATIONS

Drug produces a tranquilizer effect, and patient should be monitored for sedation effects.

metoclopramide hydrochloride (Reglan)

■ **Classification:** Antiemetic

HOW SUPPLIED/USUAL DOSAGE

IV 10 mg for adults, IV 2.5 to 5 mg for children ages 6 to 14.

OR INDICATION/COMMON USE

Usually administered IV for prevention and treatment of nausea and vomiting pre- and postoperatively.

CONTRAINDICATIONS

Should not be given to patients with known hypersensitivity, GI obstruction or hemorrhage, or a history of seizure disorders.

SPECIAL CONSIDERATIONS

Safety not established with pregnancy and lactation.

promethazine (Phenergan)

■ **Classification:** Antiemetic

HOW SUPPLIED/USUAL DOSAGE

IV 25 to 50 mg Ampule and can be given IV or IM every four to six hours as needed.

OR INDICATION/COMMON USE

Used to treat and prevent nausea and vomiting pre- and postoperatively.

CONTRAINDICATIONS

Should not be given to patients with a known hypersensitivity, prostatic hypertrophy, or narrow-angle glaucoma.

SPECIAL CONSIDERATIONS

Can be mixed with Demerol for an enhanced effect, but caution should be used as promethazine potentiates the effect of the Demerol and sedation. When promethazine is used alone it has a sedative effect in majority of patients.

ondansetron hydrochloride (Zofran)

■ **Classification:** Antiemetic

HOW SUPPLIED/USUAL DOSAGE

IV 4 mg undiluted over 2 to 5 minutes.

OR INDICATION/COMMON USE

Used to prevent postoperative nausea and vomiting.

CONTRAINDICATIONS

Should not be given to patients with known hypersensitivity.

SPECIAL CONSIDERATIONS

Can be diluted in 50 mL of D5W for IV infusion.

prochlorperazine (Compazine)

Classification: Antiemetic

HOW SUPPLIED/USUAL DOSAGE

IV 5 to 10 mg.

OR INDICATION/COMMON USE

Used for pre- and postoperative nausea control.

CONTRAINDICATIONS

Should not be given to patients with a known hypersensitivity, CNS depression such as coma, and is contraindicated in pediatric surgery.

SPECIAL CONSIDERATIONS

Drug has a sedative effect and patient should be monitored after administration.

CARDIAC MEDICATIONS

digoxin

dopamine hydrochloride (Intropin, Revimine)

nitroglycerin – glyceryl trinitrate (Nitro-Bid IV, Nitrostat IV, Nitroject, and Tridil)

nitroprusside sodium (Nipride)

norepinephrine bitartate (Levophed)

papaverine hydrochloride (Pavatine)

phenylephrine hydrochloride (Neo-Synephrine)

digoxin

■ **Classification:** Cardiac Medications (Antiarrhythmic, Cardiotonic)

HOW SUPPLIED/USUAL DOSAGE

IV loading dose 10 to 15 mcg/kg in 3 divided doses every 6 to 8 hours with the first dose equal to 50% of the total dose. Maintenance dose of 125 to 350 mcg/day every day or twice daily.

OR INDICATION/COMMON USE

Used to treat heart failure, atrial fibrillation, and atrial flutter.

CONTRAINDICATIONS

Should not be given to patients with ventricular fibrillation and ventricular tachycardia.

SPECIAL CONSIDERATIONS

Digoxin toxicity can occur at any time in dosing process.

dopamine hydrochloride (Intropin, Revimine)

■ **Classification:** Cardiac Medications (Cardiac Stimulant, Vasopressor)

HOW SUPPLIED/USUAL DOSAGE

IV infusion—0.3 to 3 mcg/kg/min for vasodilation of renal arteries; 2 to 10 mcg/kg/min for increased cardiac output. Dosage can be increased to 50 mcg/kg/min if necessary.

OR INDICATION/COMMON USE

Shock, MI, trauma, severe hypotension, and open-heart surgery.

CONTRAINDICATIONS

Should not be given to patients with uncorrected ventricular fibrillation, ventricular tachycardia, and other tachycardia arrhythmias.

SPECIAL CONSIDERATIONS

Dosage should not exceed 50 mcg/kg/min or excessive vasodilation can occur. B/P and heart rate must be constantly monitored when using dopamine hydrochloride.

nitroglycerin — glyceryl trinitrate (Nitro-Bid IV, Nitrostat IV, Nitroject, and Tridil)

■ **Classification:** Cardiac Medications (Vasodilator, Antianginal, Antihypertensive)

HOW SUPPLIED/USUAL DOSAGE

IV infusion—5 mcg/min initially, increasing 5 mcg/min every 3 to 5 minutes to 20 mcg/min, and can be increased 10—20 mcg/min every 3 to 5 minutes until desired effect occurs.

OR INDICATION/COMMON USE

To prevent angina, manage hypertension, or treat heart failure.

CONTRAINDICATIONS

Should not be given to patients with severe anemia, head trauma or increased ICP, glaucoma, hypotension, hypovolemia, constrictive pericarditis, pericardial tamponade, or a tolerance to nitrates.

SPECIAL CONSIDERATIONS

Blood pressure and heart rate should be monitored continuously during infusion therapy, and patients frequently experience headaches with nitroglycerin treatment.

nitroprusside sodium (Nipride)

■ **Classification:** Cardiac Medications (Antihypertensive, Vasodilator)

HOW SUPPLIED/USUAL DOSAGE

IV infusion—loading dose of 0.25 to 0.3 mcg/kg/min, increasing gradually to achieve desired blood pressure with a maximum dose of 10 mcg/kg/min.

OR INDICATION/COMMON USE

Used to produce controlled hypotension in vascular procedures and during the use of anesthesia.

CONTRAINDICATIONS

Should not be given to patients in acute heart failure, with decreased cerebral circulation, and hypertension from aortic coartication or AV shunting.

SPECIAL CONSIDERATIONS

Patients receiving Nipride should have blood pressure and heart rate monitored continuously.

norepinephrine bitartate (Levophed)

■ **Classification:** Cardiac Medications (Cardiac Stimulant, Vasopressor)

HOW SUPPLIED/USUAL DOSAGE

IV infusion—initially 0.5 to 1 mcg/kg/min, increasing as needed to reach desired blood pressure. Maintenance dosage—2 to 12 mcg/kg/min.

OR INDICATION/COMMON USE

Severe hypotension, cardiac arrest, shock, and sometimes spinal anesthesia.

CONTRAINDICATIONS

Should not be given to patients with hypovolemia, mesenteric, or peripheral vascular thrombosis, and when using hydrocarbon inhalation anesthesia (halothane).

SPECIAL CONSIDERATIONS

Dosage should not exceed 30 mcg/kg/min. Blood pressure and heart rate should be monitored when using Levophed.

papaverine hydrochloride (Pavatine)

Classification: Cardiac Medications (Vasodilator)

HOW SUPPLIED/USUAL DOSAGE

IM/IV dose varies, but typically is 30 to 120 mg every three hours as needed.

OR INDICATION/COMMON USE

Used in cardiac bypass surgery, as a peripheral vasodilator and to prevent vasospasms in the harvested vessels to be used for bypass.

CONTRAINDICATIONS

Should not be given to patients with complete AV block.

SPECIAL CONSIDERATIONS

Used primarily in bypass surgery to prevent vasospasms in harvested vessels by flushing the vessel, letting it soak in a papaverine solution, and flushing again before attaching the vessel for the bypass. Can be administered IV to aid in perfusion of peripheral vessels.

phenylephrine hydrochloride (Neo-Synephrine)

■ **Classification:** Cardiac Medications (Antiarrhythmic, Vasoconstrictor, Vasopressor)

HOW SUPPLIED/USUAL DOSAGE

IV infusion—100 to 180 mcg/min (0.1 to 0.18 mg) until blood pressure stabilizes. Maintenance dosage—40 to 60 mcg/min or according to patient condition.

OR INDICATION/COMMON USE

To treat hypotension or maintain blood pressure during anesthesia, and to treat vascular failure in shock.

CONTRAINDICATIONS

Should not be given to patients with severe coronary disease, severe hypertension, ventricular tachycardia, and pregnancy.

SPECIAL CONSIDERATIONS

Blood pressure and heart rate should be monitored when patients receive Neo-Synephrine.

COAGULANTS/ HEMOSTATIC AGENTS/ SEALANTS

protamine sulfate (heparin antagonist)

absorbable gelatin (Gelfoam)

microfibrillar collagen (Avitene)

oxidized cellulose (Oxycel, Surgicel)

thrombin (Thrombostat)

DuraSeal™ Spine Sealant

Floseal™ Matrix Hemostatic Sealant

Vitagel™ Surgical Hemostat

protamine sulfate (heparin antagonist)

■ **Classification:** Coagulants

HOW SUPPLIED/USUAL DOSAGE

Each mg of protamine sulfate will neutralize: 90 units of beef-lung heparin, 115 units of intestinal mucosa-derived heparin, and 100 units of calcium heparin.

OR INDICATION/COMMON USE

Antidote for heparin administration during extracorpeal circulation and other vascular procedures requiring large amounts of heparin intra-operatively.

CONTRAINDICATIONS

Should only be administered to patients that have received heparin. If patient has a hypersensitivity to protamine sulfate the symptoms of the allergic reaction are treated and the drug will continue to be used for heparin effects reversal.

SPECIAL CONSIDERATIONS

Can cause an abrupt drop in blood pressure, urticaria, pulmonary edema, and anaphylaxis.

Absorbable Gelatin (Gelfoam)

■ **Classification:** Hemostatic Agent

HOW SUPPLIED/USUAL DOSAGE

Powder form mixed with Sterile Saline to make a paste to be applied to bone.

Compressed and uncompressed pad form in various sizes can be cut or applied whole.

OR INDICATION/COMMON USE

Indicated for capillary bleeding and cancellous bone oozing. Pad is placed over bleeding capillaries, and as fibrin is deposited in the interstices the sponge swells and forms a clot.

CONTRAINDICATIONS

Should not be used when cell saver is in use.

SPECIAL CONSIDERATIONS

Agent can be left in the patient and does not have to be removed as it is absorbable.

Microfibrillar Collagen (Avitene)

■ **Classification:** Hemostatic Agent

HOW SUPPLIED/USUAL DOSAGE

Thin compressed pad form is applied directly to bleeding source in dry form and becomes an active hemostatic agent.

OR INDICATION/COMMON USE

Indicated for bleeding from raw surfaces, including bone and friable tissue, and can also be molded to fit into crevices and around suture lines.

CONTRAINDICATIONS

Should not be used when cell saver is in use.

SPECIAL CONSIDERATIONS

Agent is absorbable and can be left inside the patient. Using two sheets of Avitene with a layer of Surgicel in between on oozing surfaces is called an Avitene Sandwich and may be used with bleeding that is difficult to stop.

Oxidized Cellulose (Oxycel, Surgicel)

■ **Classification:** Hemostatic Agent

HOW SUPPLIED/USUAL DOSAGE

Pad of oxidized cellulose or knitted fabric strip, can be wrapped around structures or simply laid dry against bleeding surfaces.

OR INDICATION/COMMON USE

Agent is used for oozing and bleeding on suture lines, bone, and raw surfaces. Can be cut or used whole.

CONTRAINDICATIONS

Must be removed from bone as it will interfere with bone regeneration. Should not be used when Cell Saver is in use.

SPECIAL CONSIDERATIONS

Absorbable agent may be left in the patient, except with bone, when it should be removed.

SPECIAL CONSIDERATIONS

Thrombin (Thrombostat)

■ **Classification:** Hemostatic Agent

HOW SUPPLIED/USUAL DOSAGE

Topical form consisting of thrombin powder that is reconstituted with thrombin solution and can be applied in liquid form or used to soak Gelfoam for a more effective hemostatic reaction.

Dry thrombin powder is mixed with blood plasma and forms "fibrin glue" that is applied directly to bleeding surfaces. Thrombin spray is also available and can be sprayed directly on bleeding surfaces.

OR INDICATION/COMMON USE

Can be used alone or in conjunction with another hemostatic agent to provide more bleeding control. Gelfoam sponges are frequently soaked in thrombin for example.

CONTRAINDICATIONS

Should not be allowed to enter large blood vessels due to intravascular clotting and can result in death. Intended for capillary and venule bleeding only.

SPECIAL CONSIDERATIONS

Absorbable agent can be left inside the patient but should only be used on capillary and venule bleeding.

DuraSeal™ Spine Sealant

■ **Classification:** Spinal Sealant System

HOW SUPPLIED/USUAL DOSAGE

The DuraSeal™ Spine Sealant System is provided in two configurations. The 2 mL configuration consists of one 2 mL polymer kit and one MicroMyst™ Applicator. (The MicroMyst™ Applicator requires the use of a compressed air source, such as the Confluent Surgical Flow Regulator or the Confluent Surgical Air Pump.) The 5 mL configuration consists of one 5 mL polymer kit which includes the Dual Liquid Applicator (consisting of the Y-Applicator and three (3) Spray Tips). The polymer kits and applicators are provided sterile.

OR INDICATION/COMMON USE

Package insert states the DuraSeal™ Spine Sealant System is indicated for use as an adjunct to sutured dural repair during spinal surgery to provide a watertight closure. DuraSeal™ is NOT a hemostatic agent but instead is a dural sealant.

CONTRAINDICATIONS

Package insert states do not apply the Duraseal™ hydrogel to confined bony structures where nerves are present since neural compression may result due to hydrogel swelling. The hydrogel may swell to 50% of its size in any dimension. Do not use in patients younger than 18 years of age or in pregnant or breastfeeding females.

(continues)

DuraSeal™ Spine Sealant continued

SPECIAL CONSIDERATIONS

Package insert states to use within one hour of preparation. Do not use in combination with other sealants or hemostatic agents. Prior to the application of the hydrogel, ensure that adequate hemostasis has been achieved. Incidental application of hydrogel to tissue planes that will be subsequently approximated, such as muscle and skin, should be avoided.

Floseal™ Matrix Hemostatic Sealant

■ **Classification:** Hemostatic Agent

HOW SUPPLIED/USUAL DOSAGE

Supplied in kit form with 1—5 mL syringe with Gelatin Matrix, 1—5 mL syringe with female to female Luer connector and one bowl for thrombin. Thrombin must be added to Gelatin Matrix prior to use.

OR INDICATION/COMMON USE

Floseal is used in surgical procedures, other than ophthalmic, as an adjunct to hemostasis when control of bleeding by conventional procedures is ineffective or impractical.

Thrombin is reconstituted and supplied to sterile field per sterile technique; the thrombin is drawn into the female syringe and connected to the syringe with Gelatin Matrix. The syringes are then mixed until thrombin is absorbed into Gelatin Matrix. The mixture is ready for use and can be applied to bleeding surfaces.

CONTRAINDICATIONS

Package insert states Floseal should not be injected directly into blood vessels, should not be used on skin incisions, and should not be used in patients with allergy to material of bovine origin or thrombin.

(continues)

Floseal™ Matrix Hemostatic Sealant continued

SPECIAL CONSIDERATIONS

Package insert recommends applying direct pressure with a sponge for two minutes immediately after application of the product to bleeding surface. Floseal can remain in tissue and does not have to be removed.

Vitagel™ Surgical Hemostat

■ **Classification:** Hemostatic Agent

HOW SUPPLIED/USUAL DOSAGE

The Vitagel™ Surgical Hemostat system requires a CellPaker™ Collection Device, centrifuge, and the Vitagel™ Surgical Hemostat Delivery System (refrigerated); 10 mL of the patient's arterial or venous blood is drawn in the CellPack™ Collection Device and mixed in the centrifuge. The package instructions are then followed to prepare the delivery system for use. Package inserts states it requires five to seven minutes to prepare for use.

OR INDICATION/COMMON USE

Package insert states that Vitagel is indicated in surgical procedures (other than in neurosurgical and ophthalmic) as an adjunct to hemostasis when control of bleeding by ligature or conventional procedures is ineffective or impractical.

CONTRAINDICATIONS

Package insert states do not use in patients who have shown a sensitivity to any of the components and/or to materials of bovine origin. Do not inject into blood vessels or allow to enter blood vessels, as extensive intravascular clotting or even death may result.

(continues)

Vitagel™ Surgical Hemostat continued

SPECIAL CONSIDERATIONS

Package insert states Vitagel uses microfibrillar collagen and thrombin in combination with the patient's own plasma (fibrinogen and platelets). This combination produces an effective and safe hemostat by forming a collagen/fibrin scaffold with platelets. Vitagel has been shown to be effective in controlling bleeding during orthopaedic, cardiac, hepatic, and general surgical procedures when other hemostatic agents are not effective or able to be used.

DIURETICS

bumetanide (Bumex)

furosemide (Lasix)

mannitol (Osmitrol)

bumetanide (Bumex)

Classification: Diuretics

HOW SUPPLIED/USUAL DOSAGE

Injection 0.25 mg/mL
Dosage determined by anesthesia.

OR INDICATION/COMMON USE

Used in surgical patients to reduce edema caused by cardiac dysfunction and/or renal disease. Typically administered by anesthesia when the patient's metabolic indicators warrant use, has a rapid onset within minutes, and duration is 30 minutes to one hour.

CONTRAINDICATIONS

Should not be administered to patients with a history of hypersensitivity to bumetanide or sulfonamides, and to patients with a severe electrolyte deficiency.

SPECIAL CONSIDERATIONS

Drug will cause an increased fluid output and a Foley catheter should be inserted prior to administration, as this drug has an immediate onset and effect. Catheter will also aid anesthesia in monitoring/measuring fluid output.

furosemide (Lasix)

Classification: Diuretics

HOW SUPPLIED/USUAL DOSAGE

Injection 10 mg/mL, adult—40 mg IV over 1 to 2 minutes, then 80 mg IV in 60 to 90 minutes if needed.

OR INDICATION/COMMON USE

Used in surgical patients to reduce edema, pulmonary edema, and hypertension. Typically administered by anesthesia when patient's metabolic indicators warrant use; onset is within five minutes, with duration of two hours.

CONTRAINDICATIONS

Should not be administered to patients with a history of hypersensitivity to the drug.

SPECIAL CONSIDERATIONS

Drug will cause an increased fluid output and a Foley catheter should be inserted prior to drug administration as drug has an onset of effects in five minutes. Foley will aid anesthesia in monitoring/measuring output.

mannitol (Osmitrol)

Classification: Diuretics

HOW SUPPLIED/USUAL DOSAGE

Injection 5%, 10%, 15%, 20%, and 25%. Dosage determined by anesthesia and surgeon according to patient's weight and condition

OR INDICATION/COMMON USE

Used in surgical patients for reduction of intraocular pressure, reduction of intracranial pressure, to treat oliguria or to prevent oliguria/acute renal failure. Typically administered by anesthesia in concentration required for specific condition being treated. Dosage is determined by the patient's weight and solution to be used, and onset can vary from 15 minutes to one hour, with duration of three to eight hours. Commonly used during a Craniotomy to reduce brain edema.

Can be used in irrigating solution during TURP (Transurethral Resection of Prostate Gland), should be greater than 3.5% to prevent hemolysis. Mannitol in the irrigating solution during a TURP is used to prevent abnormal fluid retention from the procedure.

CONTRAINDICATIONS

Should not be administered to patients with a history of hypersensitivity to the drug and in those with anuria, progressive renal disease or dysfunction, or active intracranial bleeding except during Craniotomy.

(continues)

mannitol (Osmitrol) continued

SPECIAL CONSIDERATIONS

For maximum effect in intraocular surgery, should be administered 60 to 90 minutes preoperatively. Foley catheter should be inserted prior to drug administration, as drug will cause increased fluid output, and anesthesia will need to monitor the output.

DYES/CONTRAST MEDIA

Gentian violet

Indigo carmine

iodixanol (Visipaque)

iohexol (Omnipaque)

Methylene blue

Methylene Blue

■ **Classification:** Dyes

HOW SUPPLIED/USUAL DOSAGE

IV 20 mL Ampule

OR INDICATION/COMMON USE

Used for skin marking prior to skin prep as well as in urological and lymphatic surgery to ensure patency of structures.

CONTRAINDICATIONS

Should not be used in patients with known allergies to Methylene Blue.

SPECIAL CONSIDERATIONS

Caution should be taken when handling the dye, as it will stain floors, furniture, and skin if accidentally spilled. Use care when applying for skin markation as the product is a dye.

iodixanol (Visipaque)

Classification: Dyes (Contrast Media)

HOW SUPPLIED/USUAL DOSAGE

Supplied in IV with concentrations of 270 mg/mL and 320 mg/mL of organically bound iodine. Concentration level and level of dilution are dependent upon the structures being injected with contrast media and the type of radiological exam/procedure.

OR INDICATION/COMMON USE

Contrast media that is typically used in peripheral vascular/angiography surgical procedures using fluoroscopy.

CONTRAINDICATIONS

Should not be administered to patients with a known hypersensitivity to iodine.

SPECIAL CONSIDERATIONS

Typically diluted in normal saline for use with fluoroscopy.

iohexol (Omnipaque)

Classification: Dyes (Contrast Media)

HOW SUPPLIED/USUAL DOSAGE

Supplied in IV form with iodine concentration levels that include 140, 180, 240, 300, and 350 mg/mL. Concentration level and level of dilution are dependent upon the structures being injected with contrast media and the type of radiological exam/procedure.

OR INDICATION/COMMON USE

Typically the contrast media of choice for use in surgical procedures for viewing GU structures, the biliary tree to include the common bile duct, and vascular structures.

CONTRAINDICATIONS

Should not be administered to patients with a known hypersensitivity to iodine.

SPECIAL CONSIDERATIONS

Typically diluted in Normal Saline for use with fluoroscopy.

Indigo Carmine

■ **Classification:** Dyes

HOW SUPPLIED/USUAL DOSAGE

IV 5 mg ampule.

OR INDICATION/COMMON USE

Used in urological surgery to view ureteral orifices.

CONTRAINDICATIONS

Should not be given to patients with known hypersensitivity.

SPECIAL CONSIDERATIONS

Use care when handling the dye as it is royal blue and will stain tissue.

Gentian Violet

■ **Classification:** Dyes

HOW SUPPLIED/USUAL DOSAGE

Topical solution in various dosage supplies.

OR INDICATION/COMMON USE

Used to mark the skin before skin prep.

CONTRAINDICATIONS

Should not be given to patients with known hypersensitivity.

SPECIAL CONSIDERATIONS

Topical solution only, do not give IV.

HORMONES

dexamethasone acetate
(Decadron LA, Dexone LA)

insulin

dexamethasone acetate (Decadron LA, Dexone LA)

Classification: Hormones (Corticosteroid)

HOW SUPPLIED/USUAL DOSAGE

IV—8 to 16 mg for intraarticular injection.

OR INDICATION/COMMON USE

Frequently injected intra-articular through arthroscope for postoperative anti-inflammatory effect and may be combined with a local anesthetic such as Xylocaine for reduction of postoperative pain.

CONTRAINDICATIONS

Should not be given to patients with suppressed immune systems.

SPECIAL CONSIDERATIONS

May increase glucose and cholesterol levels. Diabetic patient's glucose level should be monitored every two hours after injection.

insulin (multiple brands)

■ **Classification:** Hormones

HOW SUPPLIED/USUAL DOSAGE

Supplied in rapid-acting, short-acting, intermediate-acting, long-acting, and pre-mixed forms. The form used and specific dosage is based on the patient's blood glucose level, weight, exercise, and diet. During surgery the anesthesia provider will monitor the blood glucose level during surgery and administer the form and dose required to maintain a safe blood glucose level.

OR INDICATION/COMMON USE

Most common use is by anesthesia provider to maintain a safe blood glucose level during surgery on diabetic patients.

CONTRAINDICATIONS

Insulin should not be administered in patients with a normal to low blood glucose level, as it will decrease blood glucose levels.

SPECIAL CONSIDERATIONS

Anesthesia affects the normal metabolic and physiological process of insulin, and blood glucose will need

(continues)

insulin (multiple brands) continued

to be monitored closely. Medical history with insulin form and dosage should be available on the chart prior to the induction of anesthesia in patients receiving insulin therapy.

IV FLUIDS/IRRIGATION SOLUTIONS

dextran, high-molecular weight (Dextran 75)

Glycine (1.5% Glycine Irrigation)
hetastarch (Hespan)

Ringer's Injection, lactated (Lactated Ringers Solution)

sodium bicarbonate

sodium chloride (Normal Saline)

Sorbitol (3.3% Sorbitol Irrigation)

dextran, high-molecular weight (Dextran 75)

■ **Classification:** IV Solution (Volume Expander)

HOW SUPPLIED/USUAL DOSAGE

6% dextran in Normal Saline.

OR INDICATION/COMMON USE

Plasma volume expansion in emergencies when patient has suffered extensive hemorrhage.

CONTRAINDICATIONS

Should not be given to patients with cardiac decompensation, severe oliguria, and hypervolemia.

SPECIAL CONSIDERATIONS

Anaphylactic reaction will occur early in infusion if patient is hypersensitive to the drug. Drug metabolizes to glucose and will increase blood glucose levels. It is not a replacement for blood or blood products.

Glycine (1.5 % Glycine Irrigation)

Classification: Urological Irrigation Solution

HOW SUPPLIED/USUAL DOSAGE

1.5% Glycine Irrigation is supplied in 3000 and 5000 mL plastic containers, and amount used is determined by the surgeon and surgical procedure. Each 100 mL contains 1.5 g of Glycine in water for injection.

OR INDICATION/COMMON USAGE

This solution is only used as a urologic irrigating fluid with endoscopic instruments during transurethral procedures.

CONTRAINDICATIONS

Not for injection and should only be used as urological irrigating solution. Should be used with caution in patients with severe cardiopulmonary or renal dysfunction.

SPECIAL CONSIDERATIONS

Frequently used for transurethral resection of the prostrate (TURP) and other transurethral procedures requiring the use of electrocautery.

hetastarch (Hespan)

Classification: IV Solutions (Plasma Expander)

HOW SUPPLIED/USUAL DOSAGE

6 gm/100 mL Normal Saline.

OR INDICATION/COMMON USE

Plasma expander in emergency situations.

CONTRAINDICATIONS

Should not be given to patients with severe oliguria or hypervolemia.

SPECIAL CONSIDERATIONS

Is not a replacement for blood or blood products and can be used in combination with blood and blood products.

Ringer's injection, lactated (Lactated Ringers Solution)

■ **Classification:** IV Solutions

HOW SUPPLIED/USUAL DOSAGE

150, 250, 500, and 1,000 mL.

OR INDICATION/COMMON USE

Fluid and electrolyte replacement during surgery. Given as a bolus to expand blood volume and aid in increasing blood pressure.

CONTRAINDICATIONS

Should not be given to patients in fluid or metabolic overload.

SPECIAL CONSIDERATIONS

Can be given to renal failure patients as an emergency volume expander.

sodium bicarbonate

■ **Classification:** IV Solutions

HOW SUPPLIED/USUAL DOSAGE

IV dosage dependent upon patient condition or arterial blood gases.

OR INDICATION/COMMON USE

Cardiac arrest and/or metabolic acidosis.

CONTRAINDICATIONS

Should not be given to patients in cardiac arrest unless metabolic acidosis is present.

SPECIAL CONSIDERATIONS

Arterial blood gases should be monitored when using sodium bicarbonate.

sodium chloride (Normal Saline)

■ **Classification:** IV Solutions

HOW SUPPLIED/USUAL DOSAGE

50, 100, 250, 500, 1000, and 3000 mL IV solution. Sodium solution for Normal Saline if 0.9% and ½ Normal Saline is 0.45%.

Available in bottled form, and this should not be confused with IV sodium chloride; bottled form cannot be used in the same manner as IV solution. Bottled form should be used only as an irrigant if no drugs will be added.

OR INDICATION/COMMON USE

Normal fluid replacement/fluid maintenance, and used as irrigation solution for surgical procedures.

CONTRAINDICATIONS

Should not be given to patients in fluid overload or in renal failure.

SPECIAL CONSIDERATIONS

IV solution should be used to reconstitute powder forms of drugs and if antibiotic is used in irrigation solution. Bottled form should not be used for reconstitution of drugs and/or as an irrigation solution during any vascular procedures.

Sorbitol (3.3% Sorbitol Irrigation)

■ **Classification:** Urological Irrigation Solution

HOW SUPPLIED/USUAL DOSAGE

3.3% Sorbitol Irrigation is supplied in 2000, 3000, and 4000 mL plastic containers, and amount used is determined by the surgeon and surgical procedure. Each 100 mL contains 3,3 g Sorbitol Solution in water for injection.

OR INDICATION/COMMON USE

This solution is only used as a urologic irrigating fluid with endoscopic instruments during transurethral procedures.

CONTRAINDICATIONS

Not for injection, and should only be used as urological irrigating solution.

SPECIAL CONSIDERATIONS

Frequently used for transurethral resection of the prostrate (TURP) and other transurethral procedures requiring the use of electrocautery.

NARCOTIC ANTAGONISTS

flumazenil (Romazicon)

naloxone hydrochloride (Narcan)

nalmefene hydrochloride

flumazenil (Romazicon)

Classification: Narcotic Antagonist

HOW SUPPLIED/USUAL DOSAGE

IV 0.2 mg repeated at one-minute intervals, usually 0.6 to 1 mg is effective in reversal. No more than 1 mg in a single dose, and no more than 3 mg in one hour.

OR INDICATION/COMMON USE

Complete or partial reversal of sedative effects of benzodiazepines after anesthesia or conscious sedation.

CONTRAINDICATIONS

Should not be given to patients who have received a benzodiazepine for a life-threatening condition such as status epilepticus.

SPECIAL CONSIDERATIONS

Patient should be monitored for re-sedation as the action of the drug is shorter than any benzodiazepine. Can cause dizziness, seizures, arrhythmias, nausea, vomiting, and hyperventilation.

naloxone hydrochloride (Narcan)

Classification: Narcotic Antagonist

HOW SUPPLIED/USUAL DOSAGE

IV—Opiate overdose 0.4—2 mg, postoperative opiate depression 0.1—0.2 mg.

OR INDICATION/COMMON USE

Narcotic over-dosage and complete or partial reversal of narcotic depression. Drug of choice for opioid overdose, is given primarily for respiratory depression and reversal of narcotic analgesia.

CONTRAINDICATIONS

Should not be used in patients with respiratory depression to non-opioid drugs.

SPECIAL CONSIDERATIONS

Excessive dosage can result in reversal of analgesia, increased blood pressure, hyperventilation, surgical site bleeding, and elevated partial thromboplastin time. Too rapid reversal can cause nausea, vomiting, sweating, and tachycardia.

nalmefene hydrochloride

■ **Classification:** Narcotic Antagonist

HOW SUPPLIED/USUAL DOSAGE

Initial dose: 0.25 mcg/kg IV once followed by 0.25 mcg/kg at 2 to 5 minute intervals until the desired degree of opioid reversal is obtained.

OR INDICATION/COMMON USE

Complete or partial reversal opioid drug effects, including respiratory depression induced by natural or synthetic opioids. Also administered after benzodiazepines, inhalational anesthetics, muscle relaxants, and muscle relaxant antagonists administered in conjunction with general anesthesia.

CONTRAINDICATIONS

Should not be given to patients with a known hypersensitivity.

SPECIAL CONSIDERATIONS

If no response after a cumulative dose of 1 mcg/kg administered, additional doses are unlikely to provide an effect.

NEUROMUSCULAR BLOCKING AGENTS

atracurium besylate

pancuronium bromide

rocuronium bromide (Zemuron)

succinylcholine

vecuronium bromide

atracurium besylate

■ **Classification:** Neuromuscular blocking agent (Non-depolarizing)

HOW SUPPLIED/USUAL DOSAGE

Supplied in IV form in three different strengths and amounts, with dosage based on patient's weight. Dosage is dependent upon strength and body weight, so it is individualized for each patient.

OR INDICATION/COMMON USE

Used to facilitate endotracheal intubation, as an adjunct to general anesthesia, and to provide skeletal muscle relaxation during surgery and/or mechanical ventilation.

CONTRAINDICATIONS

Should not be given to patients with known hypersensitivity and should not be administered simultaneously with other neuromuscular blocking agents.

SPECIAL CONSIDERATIONS

Enflurane and isoflurane may enhance the neuromuscular blocking action of the drug. If other muscle relaxants are used during the same procedure an antagonist effect is possible. Succinylcholine administered prior to the drug may enhance the onset and

(continues)

atracurium besylate continued

increase the depth of neuromuscular block. Atracurium besylate should not be administered until the patient has recovered from a succinycholine induced neuromuscular block.

Pancuronium bromide

■ **Classification:** Neuromuscular blocking agent (Non-depolarizing)

HOW SUPPLIED/USUAL DOSAGE

Supplied in IV form in three different strengths and amounts, with dosage based on patient's weight. Dosage is dependent upon strength and body weight so it is individualized for each patient.

OR INDICATION/COMMON USE

Used to facilitate endotracheal intubation, as an adjunct to general anesthesia, and to provide skeletal muscle relaxation during surgery and/or mechanical ventilation.

CONTRAINDICATIONS

Should not be given to patients with known hypersensitivity and should not be administered simultaneously with other neuromuscular blocking agents.

SPECIAL CONSIDERATIONS

Enflurane and isoflurane enhances the neuromuscular blocking action of the drug. If other muscle relaxants are used during the same procedure an antagonist effect is possible. Succinylcholine administered prior to the drug may enhance the onset and increase the depth of neuromuscular block. Pancuronium bromide should not be administered until the patient has recovered from a succinycholine-induced neuromuscular block.

rocuronium (Zemuron)

Classification: Neuromuscular blocking agent (Non-depolarizing)

HOW SUPPLIED/USUAL DOSAGE

Supplied in IV form in two different strengths and amounts with dosage based on patient's weight and desired effect for intubation or maintenance of relaxation. Dosage is dependent upon strength and body weight so it is individualized for each patient.

OR INDICATION/COMMON USE

Used as an adjunct to general anesthesia, to facilitate both rapid sequence and routine endotracheal intubation, and to provide skeletal muscle relaxation during surgery or mechanical ventilation.

CONTRAINDICATIONS

Should not be given to patients with known hypersensitivity and should not be administered simultaneously with other neuromuscular blocking agents. After IV administration the IV tubing should be flushed before administering other IV drugs, as several drugs are incompatible with rocuronium bromide.

SPECIAL CONSIDERATIONS

Enflurane and isoflurane will enhance the neuromuscular blocking action of the drug. If other muscle relaxants are used during the same procedure an

(continues)

rocuronium (Zemuron) continued

antagonist effect is possible. Rocuronium bromide should not be administered until the patient has recovered from a succinycholine-induced neuromuscular block.

succinylcholine

■ **Classification:** Neuromuscular blocking agent (Depolarizing)

HOW SUPPLIED/USUAL DOSAGE

Supplied in IV form, with dosage based on patient's weight and the desired effect of relaxation. Dosage is dependent upon strength and body weight so it is individualized for each patient.

OR INDICATION/COMMON USE

Used to facilitate endotracheal intubation, as an adjunct to general anesthesia, and to provide skeletal muscle relaxation during surgery.

CONTRAINDICATIONS

Succinylcholine should not be used in patients with a history or family history of malignant hyperthermia or skeletal muscle diseases. If symptoms of a malignant hyperthermia crisis develop, then the administration of the succinylcholine should be stopped immediately.

SPECIAL CONSIDERATIONS

Succinylcholine has a profound effect and induces muscle paralysis. Patients should be monitored for muscle rigidity or a rapid increase in body temperature for potential malignant hyperthermia crisis.

vecuronium bromide

■ **Classification:** Neuromuscular blocking agent (Non-depolarizing)

HOW SUPPLIED/USUAL DOSAGE

Supplied in IV form in two different strengths, with dosage based on patient's weight. Dosage is dependent upon strength and body weight so it is individualized for each patient.

OR INDICATION/COMMON USE

Used to facilitate endotracheal intubation, as an adjunct to general anesthesia, and to provide skeletal muscle relaxation during surgery and/or mechanical ventilation.

CONTRAINDICATIONS

Should not be given to patients with known hypersensitivity and should not be administered simultaneously with other neuromuscular blocking agents.

SPECIAL CONSIDERATIONS

Enflurane and isoflurane enhances the neuromuscular blocking action of the drug. If other muscle relaxants are used during the same procedure an antagonist effect is possible. Succinylcholine administered prior to the drug may enhance the onset and increase the depth of the neuromuscular block from vecuronium bromide.

OBSTETRICAL AGENTS

oxytocin (Pitocin)

oxytocin (Pitocin)

■ **Classification:** Obstetrical Agents

HOW SUPPLIED/USUAL DOSAGE

IV—1 mL (10-unit) ampule in 1000 mL of D5W, Lactated Ringers, or Normal Saline, infused at 1 to 2 milliunits/minutes. Rate is increased 1 to 2 milliunits/minutes at 15 to 30 minute intervals until normal contraction pattern is established.

OR INDICATION/COMMON USE

Most common use is to induce or stimulate labor. May also be used in conjunction with a Dilation and Curettage for incomplete abortion (miscarriage) to reduce bleeding.

CONTRAINDICATIONS

Do not give as a bolus—should be delivered in an IV piggyback infusion so the drug can be stopped without interfering with the IV line.

SPECIAL CONSIDERATIONS

May be given to promote uterine contractions to deliver the placenta and reduce postpartum bleeding.

OPHTHALMIC

acetylcholine chloride (Miochol-E)

carbachol (Miostat)—intraocular injection

carbachol (Carboptic)—topical

pilocarpine hydrochloride (Akarpine, Isopto Carpine, Micocarpine)

fluribiprofen sodium (Ocufen)

acetylcholine chloride (Miochol-E)

■ **Classification:** Ophthalmic (Miotic)

HOW SUPPLIED/USUAL DOSAGE

Ophthalmic injection—0.5 to 2 mL instilled into anterior chamber.

OR INDICATION/COMMON USE

Used during anterior segment surgery—instilled before or after sutures are secured.

CONTRAINDICATIONS

Should not be given to patients who are hypersensitive to medication or its components.

SPECIAL CONSIDERATIONS

Be alert not to confuse Acetylcholine with Acetylcysteine.

carbachol (Miostat)—intraocular injection carbachol (Carboptic)—topical

Classification: Ophthalmic (Miotic)

HOW SUPPLIED/USUAL DOSAGE

Intraocular injection—0.5 mL instilled into anterior chamber.

OR INDICATION/COMMON USE

Used to produce pupillary miosis in ocular surgery and can be instilled before or after sutures are secured.

CONTRAINDICATIONS

Should not be given to patients with hypersensitivity or in patients where cholinergic effects such as constriction are undesirable.

SPECIAL CONSIDERATIONS

Patients with dark irises (hazel and brown eyes) may require more of the injection to be instilled because eye pigment may absorb drug.

pilocarpine hydrochloride (Akarpine, Isopto Carpine, Micocarpine)

■ **Classification:** Ophthalmic (Miotic)

HOW SUPPLIED/USUAL DOSAGE

Ophthalmic solution—1 drop in affected eye.

OR INDICATION/COMMON USE

Used to reduce intraocular pressure to protect the lens during surgery and laser Iridotomy. Counteract effects of mydriatics and cycloplegia following surgery.

CONTRAINDICATIONS

Should not be used in patients with hypersensitivity to the drug or where cholinergic effects such as constriction are undesirable.

SPECIAL CONSIDERATIONS

Patients with dark irises (hazel and brown eyes) may require more of the injection to be instilled because eye pigment may absorb drug.

fluribiprofen sodium (Ocufen)

■ **Classification:** Ophthalmic (Anti-inflammatory)

HOW SUPPLIED/USUAL DOSAGE

Ophthalmic solution—two hours before surgery, instill 1 drop into affected eye every 30 minutes before surgery, for a total of 4 drops.

OR INDICATION/COMMON USE

Used to inhibit miosis during ophthalmic surgery.

CONTRAINDICATIONS

Safe use in pregnancy and breast-feeding has not been established.

SPECIAL CONSIDERATIONS

Be alert not to confuse Ocufen with Ocuflox.

SEDATIVES/HYPNOTICS

midazolam hydrochloride (Versed)

phenobarbital (Luminal)

pentobarbital (Nembutal)

secobarbital Sodium
(Seconal Sodium)

midazolam hydrochloride (Versed)

■ **Classification:** Sedative (Adjunct to General Anesthesia) (Benzodiazepine)

HOW SUPPLIED/USUAL DOSAGE

Conscious Sedation: IM 0.07–0.08 mg/kg 30–60 minutes before the procedure. IV 1–1.5 mg five minutes before the procedure.

IV Induction for General Anesthesia: 0.30–0.35 mg/kg over 20 to 30 seconds.

OR INDICATION/COMMON USE

Can be used as sedation before general anesthesia induction and for conscious sedation prior to short diagnostic and endoscopic procedures.

CONTRAINDICATIONS

Should not be given to patients with glaucoma, shock, coma, and acute alcohol intoxication.

SPECIAL CONSIDERATIONS

Commonly causes retrograde amnesia, lightheadedness, and slurred speech. Can cause hypotension, PVCs, tachycardia, coughing, dyspnea, hyperventilation, and blurred vision.

phenobarbital (Luminal)

■ **Classification:** Sedative (Barbiturate), Anti-Convulsant

HOW SUPPLIED/USUAL DOSAGE

IM/IV 100–200 mg/day.

OR INDICATION/COMMON USE

Pediatric patients as preoperative and postoperative sedation, and to treat pylorospasm in infants.

CONTRAINDICATIONS

Should not be given to patients with a history of hepatic disease, respiratory disease, and renal disease.

SPECIAL CONSIDERATIONS

Can be used in continued anxiety or tension states as a sedative. Can cause dizziness, bradycardia, hypotension, nausea, vomiting, coughing, and possible liver damage.

pentobarbital (Nembutal)

■ **Classification:** Sedative/Hypnotic (Barbiturate)

HOW SUPPLIED/USUAL DOSAGE

Hypnotic: IM 150–200 mg. Preoperative Sedation: IM 150–200 mg in 2 doses or IV 100 mg.

OR INDICATION/COMMON USE

Sedative or hypnotic for pre-anesthetic medication, induction of general anesthesia, and as an adjunct in manipulative or diagnostic procedures.

CONTRAINDICATIONS

Should not be given to pregnant patients.

SPECIAL CONSIDERATIONS

If given rapid IV can cause respiratory depression, laryngospasm, bronchospasm, apnea, and hypotension.

secobarbital sodium (Seconal Sodium)

■ **Classification:** Sedative/Hypnotic (Barbiturate)

HOW SUPPLIED/USUAL DOSAGE

Preoperative Sedative: PO 100–300 mg one to two hours before surgery.
Hypnotic: PO/IM 100–200 mg.
Adjunct to Spinal Anesthesia: IV 50–150 mg.

OR INDICATION/COMMON USE

Preoperatively to provide basal hypnosis for general, spinal, or regional anesthesia.

CONTRAINDICATIONS

Should not be given to patients with renal insufficiency or to pregnant women.

SPECIAL CONSIDERATIONS

Can cause drowsiness, lethargy, and respiratory depression.

TRANQUILIZERS

diazepam (Valium)

hydroxyzine hydruchloride (Vistaril and Vistazine)

lorazepam (Ativan)

diazepam (Valium)

Classification: Tranquilizer (Anxiolytics), Antianxiety, Anticonvulsant, Skeletal Muscle Relaxant

HOW SUPPLIED/USUAL DOSAGE

Conscious Sedation: IV—titrate dose to desired sedation, up to 20 mg or 5–10 mg IM 30 minutes before the procedure.
Preoperative sedation: IM 10 mg 30 minutes before the procedure or 10 mg IV.
Cardioversion: IV 5–15 mg 5 to 10 minutes before the procedure.
Anxiety: IM/IV 2–10 mg every 4 to 6 hours as needed.

OR INDICATION/COMMON USE

Allay anxiety and tension prior to surgery, during cardioversion and endoscopic procedures, and also as a preoperative sedative.

CONTRAINDICATIONS

Should not be given to patients in shock, coma, or with depressed vital signs.

SPECIAL CONSIDERATIONS

Produces an amnesia effect, and can be used as an anticonvulsant in status epilepticus.

hydroxyzine hydrochloride (Vistaril and Vistazine)

- **Classification:** Tranquilizer (Anxiolytics) Antianxiety

HOW SUPPLIED/USUAL DOSAGE

Anxiety and Nausea 25–100 mg every 4 to 6 hours as needed.

OR INDICATION/COMMON USE

Reduce anxiety and tension preoperatively, control nausea and vomiting, and reduce narcotic requirements pre- and postoperatively.

CONTRAINDICATIONS

Should not be given to patients with a known hypersensitivity.

SPECIAL CONSIDERATIONS

Can cause sedation, dizziness, hypotension, and a dry mouth.

lorazepam (Ativan)

■ **Classification:** Tranquilizer (Anxiolytics), Antianxiety (Benzodiazepine)

HOW SUPPLIED/USUAL DOSAGE

Premedication: IM 2–4 mg (0.05 mg/kg) at least two hours before surgery or IV 0.44 mg/kg up to 2 mg 15 to 20 minutes before surgery.

OR INDICATION/COMMON USE

Pre-anesthetic medication to produce sedation and to relieve anxiety related to surgery.

CONTRAINDICATIONS

Should not be given to patients with glaucoma, acute alcohol intoxication, and depressive disorders.

SPECIAL CONSIDERATIONS

Retrograde amnesia is a common occurrence, can cause dizziness, disorientation, hypertension or hypotension, blurred vision, nausea, and vomiting.

Generic Name Index

Trade Name Index